# THE CURANDERX TOOLKIT

# THE CURANDERX TOOLKIT

### Reclaiming Ancestral Latinx
### Plant Medicine and Rituals for Healing

## Atava Garcia Swiecicki

Heyday,
Berkeley, California

Excerpt(s) from *Woman Who Glows in the Dark* by Elena Avila RN, MSN, with Joy Parker, copyright © 1999 by Elena Avila and Joy Parker. Used by permission of Tarcher, an imprint of Penguin Publishing Group, a division of Penguin Random House LLC. All rights reserved.

Excerpts from *Red Medicine: Traditional Indigenous Rites of Birthing and Healing* by Patrisia Gonzales. © 2012 Patrisia Gonzales. Reprinted by permission of the University of Arizona Press.

Excerpt from essay by Audre Lorde, "A Burst of Light: Living with Cancer," within the collection *A Burst of Light and Other Essays*. New York: Courier Dover Publications, 2017, p. 130. Used with permission from the author's estate.

Disclaimer: This book contains general information about plants that have traditionally been used as remedies and foods. The information here, while carefully researched, is not intended to replace the advice and care of a medical practitioner. All information provided in this book is for informational purposes only. Always consult with a health care provider before taking any medication, or if you have or suspect you might have a health problem. Any application of the material set forth in this book is at the reader's discretion and is their sole responsibility.

Library of Congress Cataloging-in-Publication Data

Names: Garcia Swiecicki, Atava, author.
Title: The curanderx toolkit : reclaiming ancestral Latinx plant medicine
   and rituals for healing / Atava Garcia Swiecicki.
Description: Berkeley, California : Heyday, [2022] | Includes
   bibliographical references.
Identifiers: LCCN 2021055132 (print) | LCCN 2021055133 (ebook) | ISBN
   9781597145718 (paperback) | ISBN 9781597145725 (epub)
Subjects: LCSH: Healing--Latin America. | Healers--Latin America. | Materia
   medica, Vegetable--Latin America. | Traditional medicine--Latin America.
Classification: LCC RZ999 .S86 2022  (print) | LCC RZ999  (ebook) | DDC
   615.5098--dc23/eng/20220118
LC record available at https://lccn.loc.gov/2021055132
LC ebook record available at https://lccn.loc.gov/2021055133

Cover Art: Botanical illustrations from Köhler's Medicinal Plants. Circa 1883
Cover Design: Ashley Ingram
Interior Design and Typesetting: Ashley Ingram

Published by Heyday
P.O. Box 9145, Berkeley, California 94709
(510) 549-3564
heydaybooks.com

Printed in East Peoria, Illinois, by Versa Press, Inc.

10 9 8 7 6 5 4 3 2 1

# TABLE OF CONTENTS

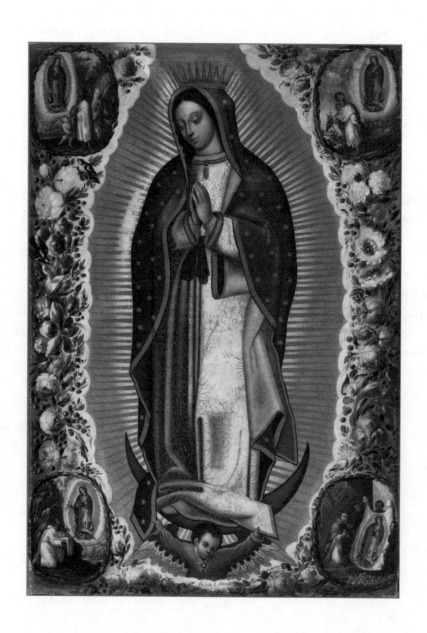

# Acknowledgments

Gratitude

First of all, I thank all the ancestors and keepers of this tradition of curanderismo, many of whom risked or lost their lives to preserve this knowledge for the past five hundred years. I thank my own ancestors who have guided me on this path of healing and remembrance. I honor the Lisjan Ohlone people and acknowledge their territory of Huchiun (Oakland), where I was blessed to be rooted for the past thirty years. Tlazohcamati to Mother Earth Tonanztin for your unconditional love, for your endless gifts, and for providing our herbal allies. Tlazohcamati to all of the extraordinary maestro/as who have guided me on this path of curanderismo: Doña Enriqueta Contreras, Estela Román, Doña Doris Ortiz, Doña Felipa Sanchez, Eleanor Barron-Druckrey, Trudy Robles, Carmen Hernandez, Maria Miranda, Lilia Román, Verónica Iglesias, Patricia Chicueyi Coatl, Cheo Torres, Laurencio López Núñez, and Sergio Magaña Ocelocoyotl.

Tlazohcamati to my mother, Julia, and my father, Michael (who is an ancestor now), for giving me the gift of life and for supporting my unconventional path, and to my sister, Jenny, who has been my lifelong companion of healing. I give thanks to my beloved companion, soul mate, and spouse, Liz Gamboa, for always having my back and for keeping me well fed and well loved. Tlazohcamati to my beloved two-spirit community for guiding me on the Red Road and being my chosen spiritual family. Tlazocamati to Danza, to all its maestros, and to all the danzantes with whom I have sweat and prayed.

Tlazohcamati to my dear friends, colleagues, and maestras who read the draft of this book and gave me their feedback: Angela Raquel Aguilar, Sandra M. Pacheco, Sara Flores, Nsomeka Gomes, Patricia Chicueyi Coatl, and Eleanor Barron-Druckrey. I give thanks for the thirteen incredible curanderx who agreed to share their stories to be included in this book. Each one of you is a bright star in the universe! Thank you for tending to your communities and being maestrx and role models for many. Tlazohcamati to Heidi Corning, Marcela Sabin, Erin Langley, and Venus Herbito, who have been cherished companions on the path of ancestral remembrance for the past two decades, and to Frances Santiago, who was the first in our circle to become an ancestor. I give thanks to all of my compañerx on this path of tending to nuestra medicina and especially to Berenice Dimas, Batul True Heart, and Melissa Reyes for saying yes and agreeing to step in to teach the Curanderx Toolkit class when I no longer could do it. I am eternally grateful for the Ancestral Apothecary community and to all our teachers and students who helped this dream of a school focused on ancestral medicine to blossom.

As a first-time author, I feel grateful to have been welcomed and supported by Heyday. Thank you to my editor Marthine Satris, for inviting me to write a book and for your guidance, kindness, and patience. Thank you to editors Michele Jones and Gayle Wattawa for your help revising the manuscript, to art director Diane Lee, and designers Ashley Ingram and Marlon Rigel for crafting a beautiful book, and to Christopher Miya and Kalie Caetano for their help with sales and marketing.

Earlier versions of portions of chapters 11, 12, and 13 appeared in a different form as "Cultivating a Healing Dream Practice" and "The Thirteen Aires and Self-Limpias" in *Voices from the Ancestors: Xicanx and Latinx Spiritual Expressions and Healing Practices*, edited by Lara Medina and Martha R. Gonzales (Tucson: University of Arizona Press, 2019). All pieces have been substantially revised and expanded for this book.

Tlazocamati to all the curanderx who humbly serve their communities across Turtle Island and are dedicated to keeping this tradition alive and vibrant. Tlazohcamati to the enduring spirit of this medicina. May it continue to thrive and grow for countless generations to come. Ometeotl!

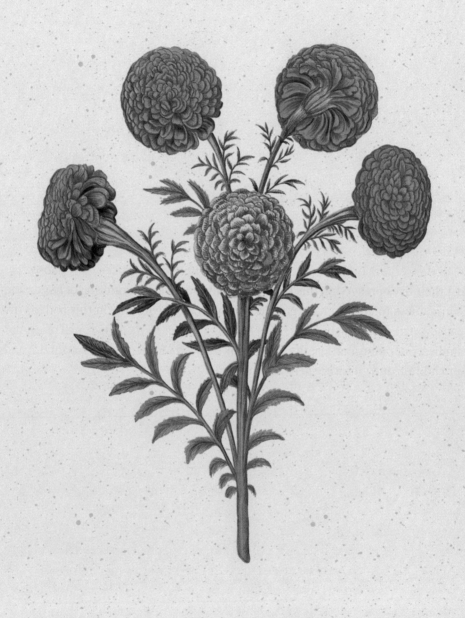

# CHAPTER 1

# Seeds

Curanderismo is not just a medical practice, but a whole culture of health.[1]

—Elena Avila

This book is a story of personal and collective healing. It is about remembering the precious knowledge that our ancestors left for us and learning how to apply that knowledge in our lives today for healing, transformation, community wellness, and social justice. This book documents a healing movement led primarily by BIPOC women, queer, trans, and nonbinary folks. It is a prayer of gratitude to all the keepers of this tradition, known and unknown, especially to those who lost their lives preserving this knowledge. My words are an offering of honor and thankfulness to all who have guided me and walked with me on this path as my teachers, friends, and students. This book is a prayer for healing for all of us, our families, our communities, the world, our beloved Mother Earth Tonantzin, and our children and all future generations.

This book began as a class I offered at Ancestral Apothecary School in Oakland, California (Huchiun, Lisjan Ohlone territory) called the Curanderx Toolkit.* As a mixed-race person of multiple ancestral lineages, I have spent all of my adult life on a quest to remember the healing traditions of my ancestors. I have dedicated time to each of my ancestral lines, yet my Mexican ancestors were the first to beckon me home.** Although because of assimilation I did not grow up with any Mexican healing traditions in my immediate family, my ancestors guided me to remember

---

* Originally the class was called the Curandera's Toolkit, but the name evolved to be more inclusive of nonbinary, gender nonconforming, and transgender people.
** Since that time, I have also spent much time working with my Polish ancestors. It is important to me to give space to all my ancestors, which is, of course, a lifetime of work.

and reconnect to their herbs, foods, rituals, and ways of praying. Through my own experience as a clinical herbalist and my studies with different curanderas and curanderos, I was eventually called to create a class on herbal medicine and healing that was grounded in the traditional medicine practices of Mexico. I dreamed that this class would be a space for collective learning, sharing, healing, and remembering ancestral medicine.

In the United States, many herbal schools teach primarily from a white European/American perspective, which is informed by western medicine and a biomedical approach to herbs. This approach to herbalism is part of my training and has value, yet I found it curious that although the United States has many communities of color with rich traditions of herbal medicine, they are not often represented in herbal education. For example, in California we have a huge Latinx population, yet very few spaces to learn about the traditional medicine of Mexico and Latin America.

*Curanderismo* can be broadly defined as the "way of healing" and refers to the traditional Indigenous and folk medicine ways of the Latinx diaspora. This includes Mexico, Central and South America, the southwestern United States, and

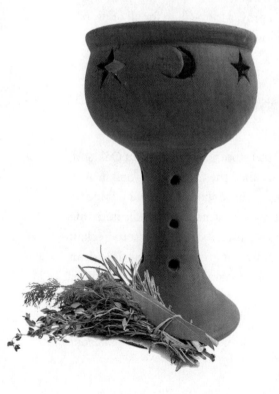

places in the Caribbean. In Mexico, curanderismo has roots in cultural practices of people from the Americas, Africa, and Europe, who all converged in early Mexico after Spanish colonization. For five hundred years, curanderismo has been primarily an oral tradition, which was never codified or standardized. Curanderismo has been primarily practiced in the home, and knowledge was passed on between family members or between teacher and student. In many places, the local curandero was the community's primary source of health care. There is no singular "curanderismo," but instead there are many ways this cultural healing system is interpreted and practiced. Curanderismo has evolved over the centuries and continues to be a very dynamic tradition.

The word *curanderismo* is a recent term that did not originate in Mexico. When I asked curandera Estela Román, she said that the term curanderismo hasn't been used historically in Mexico as a term to refer to Mexican traditional medicine. In Mexico, people call their cultural medicine practices "medicina tradicional," "medicina ancestral," or, as Maestra Estela says, "nuestra medicina." Author and partera Patrisia Gonzales calls it "Mexican traditional medicine," and she uses the term "Red Medicine" to acknowledge the similarity of Indigenous practices on both sides of the US-Mexico border.[2] I was able to track down the possible origins of the word curanderismo when I interviewed Dr. Eliseo "Cheo" Torres from the University of New Mexico. Dr. Torres has been involved in the movement to bring more attention and respect to Mexican traditional medicine since the 1960s. When I interviewed him, he said he began using the word curanderismo in the late 1980s as a way to refer to the art of traditional medicine of Mexico, because he couldn't find any other term to describe it.[3] Eventually the word made its way into the common lexicon in the United States, Mexico, and Latin America.

## Mi Camino/My Path

As theirs are for most people, my early twenties were a time of tumultuous change and growth. I had recently come out as queer, had fallen in love with my first girlfriend, and suffered a devastating breakup. My journey to understand both my queer and racial identities led me to a spiritual community led by queer and two-spirit Indigenous, Black, and Latinx women and nonbinary folks. Many of my elders in this community were people connected to their Indigenous ancestral practices, but through a queer lens. When I began to study herbal medicine, I became curious about the healing traditions of my own ancestors. My Mexican, Polish, Hungarian, and Diné (Navajo) ancestors all have rich healing traditions, yet as I grew up, I didn't learn anything about our cultural healing practices. Like many children of immigrants and detribalized Indigenous people, my grandparents and parents had assimilated to American culture, stopped speaking their mother tongues, and eventually lost many of their cultural practices. I spent much time mourning what had been apparently lost in my family line, and prayed that I could find a way to reconnect to healing traditions of my own ancestors.

In 1999, my prayers were answered when I was working at the Scarlet Sage, an herb store in San Francisco (Yelamu Ohlone territory). One day a woman walked into the store who had a strong, commanding presence. She had brown skin and long black hair streaked with gray, and was dressed in a colorful huipil. As this powerful Indigenous woman strolled through the store, she pointed to jars of dried herbs from the shelves and lectured us in Spanish about each one. I was enchanted by her presence and impressed by her knowledge.

I learned that this woman was Doña Enriqueta Contreras, a Zapotec curandera from Oaxaca, Mexico. She was a world-renowned curandera who had a vast knowledge of medicinal plants and was also a partera (midwife) who had facilitated over two thousand home births. At that time, Doña Enriqueta was traveling regularly to the United States to share her knowledge and to offer healings to the community. The moment I met Doña Enriqueta, I knew she was to be my teacher, my maestra. Even though my knowledge of Spanish was limited, I decided to become her student. I attended all the classes that she taught in Huchiun/the Bay Area, and eventually traveled down to Oaxaca to work as her apprentice.

Through Doña Enriqueta, a few months later I met another important person on my path, Mexican curandera Estela Román. At that time, Estela was the apprentice of Doña Enriqueta and accompanied her in her travels to the United States to assist her. Estela Román is from Temixco, Mexico, which is outside Cuernavaca in the state of Morelos. She comes from a family of curanderas and also had apprenticed with many of the elder curanderos in her community. Estela ran a school in Cuernavaca, where she taught the traditional medicine of Mexico.

In 2000, I traveled to Mexico to begin my formal study of curanderismo with Estela in Cuernavaca. Afterward, we traveled together down to Oaxaca to visit Doña Enriqueta, where I remained for a month to live and work with her. During the time that I learned many lessons about curanderismo, the most important was that the life of a curandera was 100 percent hard work and selfless dedication. People were knocking on Doña Enriqueta's door day and night requesting her services. In addition to offering her herbal medicine consultations, limpias, temescal ceremonies, and pregnancy and postpartum support, Doña Enriqueta also kept an immaculately clean house and provided home-cooked Oaxacan meals to everyone who stopped by her home.

Doña Enriqueta was strict and had impeccable standards for taking care of her home and her clients. I struggled to keep up with her pace and to uphold her standards. Even though I was thirty years younger than she, living day to day with Doña Enriqueta left me exhausted. She had a firm manner and did not hold back on her criticism of my performance. Sometimes our interactions left me in tears.

Twenty years later, I look back at this experience with different eyes. I understand that Doña Enriqueta was not trying to be unduly hard on me but was teaching me an important lesson about the amount of inner fortitude needed to be a curandera. I think she was also challenging me to see whether I was really dedicated to this path, or whether I was just simply trying it out. Doña Enriqueta's style of teaching is definitely old school, and she imparted lessons that were trial by fire. This kind of teaching style, although common in the Indigenous world, might be judged by western standards as being too harsh. Yet this experience was exactly what I needed to grow on my own path as a healer.

# The Path of a Curanderx

> If this your calling, it is a tremendous joy to be of service in this way. Holding space and helping others to find their way, reclaim lost part of themselves, and healing their ancestral lines is so rewarding and contributes to this time of shift for future generations and our beloved Mother Earth.
> —Brenda Salgado

Before living with Doña Enriqueta, I had a more romanticized vision of the life of a curandera. I was enamored by the glamour of the practice and a curandera's seemingly magical healing powers. Yet I realized quickly that the path of a curanderx was a path of love, self-sacrifice, and devotion to one's community. I was humbled by the experience of living with her as an apprentice and knew that if this was a path that I chose to follow, it would not be easy.

Curanderismo is a system of healing rooted in Indigenous practice and philosophy. In this tradition, the way of coming to knowledge is very different than that within a western academic paradigm. One does not become a curanderx by simply taking a class on curanderismo or by attending a weekend workshop. One is not entitled to become a curanderx by simply having the money to pay for training. The title of curanderx can never be bought. Instead, the status of curanderx is an honor bestowed by one's community as a recognition of one's gifts and service.

Some people are called to curanderismo because they are born with healing gifts, which in this tradition is called *el don*. Someone's *don* may be their healing hands, their ability to work with medicinal herbs, their beautiful singing voice, or their talent to receive messages from dreams. Often these gifts are passed on through the family bloodline, and sometimes they simply arise in a new generation. A child raised in a family that recognizes their gift may be blessed by support and mentorship from the elders in their family. This young person may be chosen to assist the curandero in their family, whether it is their abuela, tía, or parent.

Some of us were not fortunate enough to have an elder mentor in our own family. Often this is due to the impact of colonization, immigration, and assimilation, all of which cause a break in the continuation of cultural healing traditions in the family. In this case, a person may find a teacher or mentor outside their family. Yet finding a maestra or mentor is only the first step on this path. An important part of the path is for the student to demonstrate their commitment to their teacher and to the medicina itself. This demands years of dedication and service.

My initial training spanned over thirteen years, although it continues to this day more than twenty years later. After I returned from my first visit to Mexico studying with Estela Román and Doña Enriqueta Contreras, for many years I continued to learn from both of my maestras when they visited Huchiun/the Bay Area and I assisted them in their work. During this time, I learned that the work of an apprentice curanderx is selfless and requires much personal sacrifice. We learn to be of service to our maestras and to our communities. We must work hard, but at the same time remain quiet in the background. This instills humility, which is one of the most important values in curanderismo.

For those of you called to walk this path, I recommend that you begin with the search for a mentor. Start with your own family. Do you have relatives who know remedios or whom others consult for healing advice? Often these people don't even use the title of curandera/curanderx; they are simply known in their community as the person who does healings. In the past and still in many communities today, curanderas/curanderx do not advertise. They don't have websites or social media accounts. Yet people in the community know who they are and how to find them when they need help.

If you don't have people in your family to learn from, begin to explore your community. There may be an elder in your neighborhood who carries healing knowledge. Offer to help them with their daily tasks, such as shopping or weeding their garden. It takes time and work to build a relationship and to earn trust and respect.

As interest in curanderismo has grown, so have the places that offer classes or workshops. However, this is a lifelong path; there is no shortcut to learning this medicina, and attending a workshop does not make you a curanderx. What can be gained by taking classes is the knowledge to apply the practices of curanderismo for your own health and healing. Many of the practices of curanderismo can be used to take care of yourself, your family members, and your loved ones. This was the inspiration for the Curanderx Toolkit class. I wanted to teach people basic practices of curanderismo, such as making herbal teas or baños, which folks could use to support their own physical, emotional, and spiritual health.

If you are feeling called to this path and don't know where to begin, start by saying a prayer and making an offering to your own ancestors. Ask your ancestors for support and guidance. Ultimately this path is about your relationship to yourself, to your ancestors, to the Divine, and to Mother Earth Tonantzin Tlalli Coatlicue.* If you are truly called to this path, your sincere efforts will be rewarded, and opportunities to learn will open up for you.

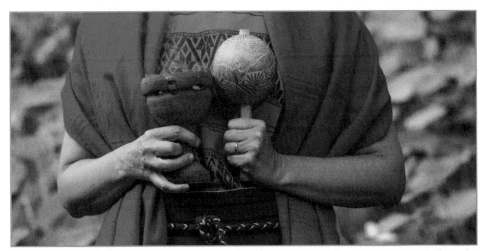

Photo by Vaschelle André

---

* Tonanztin Tlalli Coatlilcue is one name for Mother Earth in Nahuatl; she also corresponds to La Virgen de Guadalupe. In this book I will often shorten her name to Tonantzin.

# Community of Healers

As I continued to study curanderismo, I began to dream about a class that would teach herbal medicine and healing, but from a perspective of Mexican curanderismo. To bring a variety of perspectives to the class, I decided to invite local curanderas to be guest teachers so that they could present about their specialties in curanderismo. The first Curandera's Toolkit class took place in fall 2011 and over the years has become a space to nurture the growing curanderx community in Huchiun/the Bay Area, and many of the people who have contributed to the class are featured in this book.

One of the most important aspects of the curanderismo movement is the focus on building community. We are a community of healers, and all of us are responsible for preserving this medicine and walking with it in a good way. Our strength is not only in our numbers but also in our ability to collaborate on projects and to support one another. Many of us have worked together in many capacities, including organizing workshops, hosting curanderas from Mexico, and holding free community healing clinics.

Our communities are suffering, and there is a great demand for what curanderismo offers. I have received countless requests to support people after personal or collective tragedies. Curanderx are called on for support when people are sick or have suffered accidents or injuries. Curanderx are called to care for people who have lost loved ones or to help communities that have been affected by violence. Curanderx were present to help people after the California wildfires, and they offered services to immigrants detained at the border. When there is a need for healing in the community, curanderx are called on. I think it takes a village of curanderx to meet this growing need.

Also, what I have witnessed is that today curanderx are filling an important niche in the health care of our communities. Often it is the curanderx who are attending to the emotional and spiritual needs of marginalized people and communities. The curanderx whom I know are offering their services to communities of color, to people who are poor, houseless, undocumented, transgender, or recent immigrants to this country.

# Intentions for This Book

We need to leave some tools, a road map for the generations to come.

—Maria Miranda

The Curanderx Toolkit class is part of a greater resurgence of interest in curanderismo across California and across Turtle Island. More people are reclaiming their ancestral medicine and offering their healing gifts to the world. More community clinics are popping up where curanderx are offering their services. Countless people have worked hard to keep these practices alive in their communities and have contributed in a significant way to this movement.

Curanderismo is a vast body of knowledge, and in this book I cannot pretend to represent all of this tradition. Although there are common practices within curanderismo, there are also many varieties of practices and perspectives. I can only represent my own ancestral practices and the teachings that have been passed on to me by my maestras.* As I lived in California when I immersed myself in this tradition, I became part of the community of California curanderx who learn from one another and work together. Each member of this community has their own unique background and story about how they began to practice curanderismo. I will share the stories of different curanderx who have touched my life and heart, so that you may understand this system of healing from many different viewpoints. I also acknowledge that there are many curanderx in California whose stories are not included in this book.

This book covers a brief history of Mexican curanderismo, highlighting some of the herbal history. I will introduce some of the foundational theories and practices of curanderismo and the ancestral cosmovision that informs it. As I am an herbalist, much of the focus of this book is on herbal medicine. I will share how to build relationship with plants and how to discover your herbal ally, and will introduce you to some of my favorite plants to grow in gardens. I will share herbal medicine-making practices and recipes and teach you how to work

---

\* I asked for and received permission from my primary maestras to share in this book the information that they taught me.

with herbs for self-limpias and baños. We will explore the world of dreams and learn simple exercises for building your own dream practice. My intention for this book is to share the basic elements and practices of curanderismo that anyone can learn and apply to their lives.

When I wrote this book, the top principle that guided me was that I must write from my own experience. Also, I must continue in my daily life to engage with all that I am writing about. I have been on a quest for the past three decades to recover the lost fragments of my ancestral tradition. I have been taught by the plants, by los aires, by my dreams and my ancestors. Over time, I have been blessed with many maestras and maestros, each of whom carried different wisdom teachings of the tradition. I applied what I learned from my teachers to my own life. I worked with la medicina to help myself through loss, death of loved ones, grief, and many challenges. I faced two life-threatening illnesses, including uterine cancer. Time and time again la medicina of curanderismo took care of me. This book is my own road map based on the way I worked with these practices to face my personal challenges, as well as what I learned working with my students and clients. The knowledge to be gained on this path is endless. I will be a student of this tradition for the rest of my life.

I once had a dream of a sacred energy, in the form of a magical fairy-like woman who lived in the temescal of my maestra Estela Román. The message of the dream was clear: la medicina of curanderismo is alive and has a spirit. It exists beyond any human being, and it does not belong to anyone. Those of us who are fortunate to walk with this sacred energy in our lifetime have a responsibility to care for it, to bring our own contribution to it, and to pass it on to future generations. I pray that this book will plant seeds of inspiration in your heart and blossom in your consciousness. Together we can nourish this sacred gift from our ancestors and bring it forth into the world.

## Types of Curanderx

There are as many different kinds of curanderismo as there are curanderx. As I noted earlier, while practitioners of curanderismo share many common philosophies and practices, each curanderx brings their own unique flavor to their healing work. Curanderismo allows space for creativity, as well as for each healer's unique gifts and family medicine to shine and come through. What unites all practitioners of curanderismo is the connection to our cultural and ancestral healing practices and beliefs.

Within curanderismo, healers may have their own areas of expertise. Some specialists within curanderismo include parteras (midwives), sobadoras (body-workers), hueseras (bone setters), and temescaleras (leaders of temescal cere-monies). According to Elena Avila, a *curandera total* has mastered all four levels of medicine, which include teaching, bodywork, herbal medicine, and working with sacred tools such as the obsidian mirror.[4]

Today, many people practice elements of curanderismo, but not all curand-erx are at the same level of knowledge, expertise, and commitment. Curanderas such as Doña Enriqueta and Estela Román are highly skilled and are well known and respected in their communities as healers. Their healing work is their pri-mary passion, and they live their lives in service to their communities. By con-trast, many Latinx people practice elements of curanderismo in their homes with their families and loved ones, although they do not call themselves curanderx.

Many healers I know have much knowledge and experience, but do not call themselves curanderx. Some do not resonate with the name curandera ("that was just a label they put on us"),[5] and for others, that is not a term that was used traditionally in their family to describe their medicine work.[6] For still others, it feels boastful and inappropriate to assume the title of curanderx. In my perspec-tive, the title of curanderx is not one an individual chooses for themselves, but a title bestowed by one's community. The community recognizes the healer and their service to the community and honors them with the title curanderx.

## Respect for This Tradition

Although this book teaches aspects of curanderismo, this book is not a training manual to become a curanderx. The knowledge shared in this book is intended to use for yourself and your loved ones. To work as a curanderx in your commu-nity takes much more time and training beyond the scope of any book. Much of curanderismo cannot be learned in books but only through direct experience with one's teacher. It requires years of mentorship before offering one's services to the community.

Also, for those of you who do not have an ancestral connection to these traditions, please be mindful to respect this knowledge. I am sharing what I have learned because I believe that curanderismo offers something that can greatly benefit the world. I am following the lead of my teachers, who have shared this knowledge freely with people from many backgrounds. If these are not your ancestral cultural practices, I hope that what you learn in this book will inspire you to look more deeply into the healing practices of your own ancestors.

# Medicine for the Soul

> Curanderos believe that it is not enough to just heal the body. One must heal the wounded soul as well.[7]
>
> —Elena Avila

At this time in human history, we are facing the impact of centuries of capitalism, colonization, racism, and genocide. Each day, we hear more news about the destruction of the earth and the catastrophic threats to our environment from climate chaos. These events daily impact our mental, emotional, and physical health. People are yearning for ways of healing that not only treat their physical bodies but also nourish the needs of their hearts and souls.

Doña Enriqueta would often tell me that in Mexico she frequently treated illnesses in people that were the result of poverty and lack of resources. Yet when she traveled to the United States, she most often treated people who suffered from soul sickness. She said that soul sickness was an epidemic here in the US, especially for those who have had to leave their homelands to immigrate to this country.

Soul sickness can occur when we become disconnected (usually by experiencing a trauma) from our sacred body, our heart, dreams, sexuality, creativity, or spirituality. A disconnection from our roots of family, culture, ancestors, or homeland can result in soul sickness. We can suffer from soul sickness when we forget how to live in balance with Mother Earth Tonantzin. Excessive materialism, greed, and a general lack of spiritual connection can cause soul sickness. Capitalism, racism, sexism, white supremacy, homophobia, transphobia, and xenophobia all cause soul sickness. It can manifest as depression, anxiety, addiction, mental illness, or pain or disease in the physical body.

As a system of healing that grew on the blood-soaked soil of genocide and colonization, curanderismo specializes in ways to treat and heal trauma. As Avila writes, "There was a need to develop a medicine that could heal the pain and the immense susto, soul loss that resulted from the cultural destruction, enslavement and rape that occurred during the Spanish Conquest of the Americas."[8] In curanderismo, we have practices such as limpias, baños, and the temescal to help call the soul back home into the body. These practices call the soul back home by engaging all five senses. Altars adorned with colorful flowers. Aromatic bundles of rosemary or sage. Heat, steam, and sweat. Pungent copal smoke. Fragrant herbal tea and sweet chocolate. The gentle touch of loving hands. The heartbeat of the drum. By engaging all our senses, we reawaken to the splendor of life. The vibrancy of color, sound, and smell guide the lost soul back home to its sacred vessel called the body. Our herbs and flowers, as medicine of the earth, help us remember our connection to Tonantzin, the source of all life, who in turn helps heal us.

Curanderismo gives personal and intimate care to each individual and contains the most important ingredient of healing, which is love. People of many backgrounds are drawn to the practices of curanderismo because they crave a method of healing that is based in love and care and that treats the wounded soul. This book is an offering to all the people who are seeking this kind of healing, especially those of you for whom this is your ancestral medicine. My hope is that these stories inspire you to learn more, to talk with your abuelas and tías, or whoever in your family is the keeper of this knowledge. May these words help awaken your own ancestral memories.

# A Note about Language

Today, language is transforming to be more inclusive of people who identify as gender nonconforming, nonbinary, or transgender. In English, "they/them" pronouns are often used to replace "he/him" or "she/her." In Spanish, the gendered suffixes of "a" or "o" are being replaced with "e," "x," or even "@" to be gender inclusive. In the beginning, this class was called the Curandera's Toolkit, but over the years the name has transformed into the Curanderx Toolkit. In this book, I will most often use the term *curanderx* and *they/them* pronouns to refer to practitioners of curanderismo. However, when referring to many of my maestras and maestros, I will use "curandera" or "curandero," as these are the words they use to identify themselves.

This book is written in English because I am not a fluent Spanish speaker and speak little Nahuatl. As much as possible I have included words for plants in both Spanish and Nahuatl. All the different Indigenous groups of Mexico also have names for these plants in their own languages, although they are not all included in this book.* When talking about the cosmovision of the Nahua/Mexica people, I will use Nahuatl words. When referring to traditional healing concepts in curanderismo, such as susto or aires, I will use Spanish.

When talking about the cultural groups of ancient central Mexico, I will use the term *Anahuacan* instead of the anthropological word *Mesoamerican*. *Anahuac* is a Nahuatl word that refers to the central Valley of Mexico, and Anahuacan refers to the people who inhabit that region. According to Mexica and Toltec teachings, Anahuac territory encompasses land from Alaska to Nicaragua.[9]

Finally, to describe geographic locations, I am choosing to use the names of place, land, or territory used by the people indigenous to that land. To begin with, the United States was named by European colonizers, many of whom stole land from Native Americans. I will often choose the term *Turtle Island*, which is often used by North American Indigenous people, or the term *North America*, which describes the continent. All places on this continent are originally Indigenous territories and have names in the language of the native inhabitants. I acknowledge that "California" is a colonial name, but for clarity will use it when I describe this state.** I will also include the colonial names for places such as Los Angeles or Oakland to help orient readers who may not yet know the Indigenous names for these places.

---

* To look up more names for plants in Indigenous languages of Mexico, I recommend the Biblioteca Digital de la Medicina Tradicional Mexicana, http://www.medicinatradicionalmexicana.unam.mx/index.html.

** Before the Spanish invaded what we now call California in 1769, it was inhabited for thousands of years by over two hundred tribes of Indigenous people. Native California people have suffered brutal colonization, enslavement, missionization, and genocide, and their struggle to resist colonization continues today.

# Medicine for Resilience

While I was in the middle of writing this book, the entire world was turned upside down due to the COVID-19 global pandemic. In the United States, we have suffered a devastating loss of life and jobs, and many people have lost their housing. The pandemic has exposed the great inequities in health care, as Black, Indigenous, and Latinx communities have been impacted disproportionately. The combined factors of racism, social inequity, and lack of access to health care have created higher rates of both COVID-19 infection and mortality in these communities. We have witnessed too many examples where the most vulnerable members of our communities are overlooked and disregarded by government and health care during this pandemic.

In the early days of the pandemic, not only did toilet paper quickly disappear from the shelves of grocery stores, but so did any herbal medicine that treated viruses or the symptoms of COVID-19. I realized that when we are dependent on outside sources for our medicine, those sources can quickly vanish. This disappearance of medicines of all kinds has played out often in times of natural disaster, such as after Hurricane Maria in Puerto Rico. What can we do to prepare ourselves for these disasters that are inevitable due to climate crisis?

The intention of this book is to encourage you to build relationship with plants so that you have many herbal allies to support you and your loved ones in the circumstances of daily life as well as in times of crisis. The intention is also to empower everyone to grow their own herbs and to learn how to use these plants as medicine. When our medicine is growing in our communities, much of what we need will already be available in our gardens when the next natural disaster or pandemic occurs.

Curanderismo is a tradition rooted in people's resilience, and the surge of interest in curanderismo in the United States is coming at a crucial time. The ancestors of this tradition are calling many of us to remember these practices so that we can learn to be more resilient in the face of hardship and trauma. The intention of this book is to be a resource for our collective healing. My prayer is that the words I share may inspire all called to a healing path to work together to support one another, our families, and our communities through these challenging and transformative times.

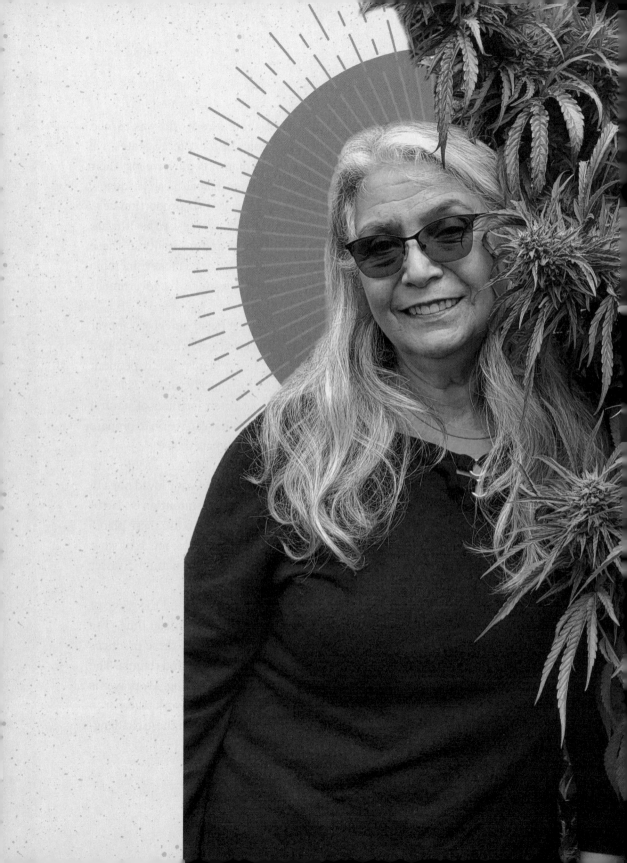

# SPOTLIGHT

# Trudy Robles
## (she/her/ella)

> "The seed of curanderismo was planted in me as a girl, and nurtured by the community who had trust and confidence in me."

Trudy Robles reminds me of the plant ruda, which is one of her primary plant allies. Like ruda, Trudy is strong, fierce, loving, and protective. I met Trudy many years ago when she helped host the first workshop taught by Estela Román in Sacramento/Nisenan territory. We shared a passion for our ancestral medicine, became fast friends, and have continued to work together over the years. Trudy is a danzante, sahumadora, promotora, and one of the founders of the monthly educational Curanderismo Series at Sol Collective, an organization dedicated to art, culture, education, activism, and wellness.

Trudy always has had "a love affair with gardening, growing plants, and making medicine." She was born and raised in Sacramento/Nisenan territory as the daughter of Mexican immigrants. Trudy grew up in an extended community of families who shared adjacent lots and who primarily lived off the land. Her family, in her words, "took their communities and their way of living in Mexico and plopped them down on the land that we grew up on in Sacramento." They had vegetable gardens and fruit orchards, and raised chickens, turkeys, goats, and cows for meat. She remembers, "We grew all our own food and canned everything, peaches, pears, chili, and sauces." Trudy's mother, Josefina, was an independent woman and a "feminist for her time." Her father, Salvador, was an avid gardener, fisherman, and hunter. He taught Trudy how to save and take care of seeds, and how to respect the elements of nature.

Trudy's Abuelo Guadalupe and her Tía Angela "had the most profound impact on my awareness of natural healing and remedios." Both were sought out by people in their community for healing. Guadalupe was a huesero, or bodyworker, who also grew lush gardens of roses, magueys, olive trees, nopales, and all kinds of herbs. "It was like paradise," Trudy recalled. Her abuelo had shelves stocked with all kinds of herbal remedios such as cannabis or romero infused in alcohol, which he would administer to all the people who came to see him for treatments. A partera and curandera, Tía Angela would treat sick or injured members of her community with teas, poultices, or other remedios. She grew herbs to use for food or medicine and was always tending to the small fire she kept behind her house, which fascinated Trudy as a child.

When I asked Trudy about her role as a curandera in the community, she responded, "A lot of my participation was birthed out of necessity." Inspired and informed by her tía's work with the fire, in the 1990s Trudy began hosting monthly full-moon fire circles for women, called lunadas. During the lunadas, women would gather to share their stories and challenges. These lunadas became important spaces for support and self-empowerment for women in the Sacramento Latinx community. Trudy recalls, "We would get together around fires. Women wanted to get out of the house and away from family and do something for themselves. We started talking about self-care and healing and our own well-being. We talked about oppression and would support one another." The lunadas started as small groups but grew considerably in size as women started to invite their friends and daughters.

Trudy credits Estela Román for being the spark that catalyzed her community's interest in ancestral medicine. Estela first traveled to Sacramento/Nisenan territory to conduct a temescal for Trudy's daughter's coming-of-age ceremony. "Estela was the fire; when she came here, she ignited us. We were already rebirthing this experience as women, but Estela's teaching ignited a fire for everyone."

Trudy also has been a leader, guiding light, and healing force in her community. She was trained by Estela to conduct the temescal ceremony for her family and community. Trudy worked for years as a sahumadora and trained dozens of young sahumadorx to work with the sacred fire and also how to work with herbs in ceremony and in healing. Trudy dedicated years of her life to organizing curanderismo classes and workshops, hosting curanderos from Mexico so that her community would have access to their ancestral knowledge and healing.

TRUDY ROBLES SPEAKS:

Love is the key.

Create space and time for self-care.

Be accountable for your own healing and actions. Choices matter—they have infinite consequences.

Be the best version of yourself. Be honest with yourself and others.

Find and connect with your spiritual self; build spiritual muscle. Listen to your spiritual self; follow the guidance, and you'll find it will make sense.

Harvest and share your wisdom.

Create your sanctuary.

Privilege and responsibility go hand in hand.

Be your own best friend, mother, sister, advocate, healer, and lover.

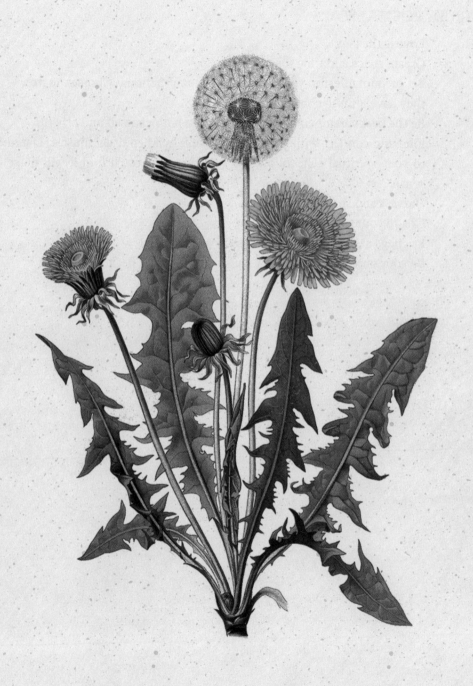

# CHAPTER 2

# Roots and Flowers

For many of our communities that have been impacted by the colonial project, these practices had to be forgotten, hidden away, or guised because of fear of persecution. Some of these practices exist in families as just ways of life or something we "just do" without that acknowledgment of our deep historical connection to the earth and a wisdom of knowing how to tend to our health at home. While I understand that these practices get categorized as "curanderismo," for me, these practices are beyond that terminology. They are live, breathing generational memory. They are resilience in the flesh. They are the conocimiento and wisdom that have survived generations of colonialism.

—Berenice Dimas

## Curanderismo in Mexico

In Mexico,* curanderismo is rooted in the practices of Indigenous people of Mexico, yet it flowered into something new as people and cultures from three continents (Africa, Europe, and the Americas) came together. It relates to the history of the colonization, resistance, and resilience of people indigenous to Mexico and Africa. Although the Spanish colonizers made calculated efforts to destroy and eradicate all the traditional healing knowledge of the Indigenous people of Mexico, our traditional medicine has persisted for five hundred years. In spite of the horrors of the transatlantic slave trade, people of African descent living in Mexico managed to preserve and practice their cultural medicine, which has had a great influence on curanderismo. As the Spanish colonized Mexico, many of their beliefs about medicine as well as medicinal plants imported from

---

* *Mexico* is a Nahuatl word that is translated to "place of the navel of the moon"; the name pre-dates Spanish colonization. This land was also called Anahuac, which translates to "land next to the water," and often refers to the central valley of Mexico.

Europe were woven into Mexican traditional medicine. In the United States/ Turtle Island, curanderismo also has a complex and multilayered history that relates to colonization, war, occupation, shifting borders, immigration, assimilation, the Chicano civil rights movement, and other forms of resistance by Latinx people.

Hundreds of years before the arrival of the Spanish colonizers, Indigenous people throughout Mexico had developed highly sophisticated systems of medicine, including vast knowledge of medicinal plants. To write about the history of each Indigenous group in Mexico is beyond the scope of this book. I will share some history of the native inhabitants of central Mexico, called the Aztec, Mexica, or Nahua people, which is the history that has been most shared with me by my maestras and maestros, many of whom come from that region. When writing about the history of Turtle Island, I am also focusing on the history of people and communities closest to me, whose legacy has directly blessed my own path.

I do not want to write about this history in a dissociative way. I cannot separate my mind from my heart and the piercing grief and burning rage I feel when reading about the senseless brutality of the "conquest" of Mexico,* or about the horrors of the transatlantic slave trade. I am burning copal and saying prayers as I write so that I may do so in a way that honors the ones who were murdered and the knowledge that was lost. My words are a prayer for healing for all of our ancestors. I am praying for the ones who were killed as well as the murderers. All of these ancestors live inside me.

Before you continue to read, I invite you to take a deep breath. Take a moment to ground yourself and feel your connection to Tonantzin. Light a candle in memory of the lives that were brutally stolen in the three hundred years of the transatlantic slave trade. Burn some copal to honor those lives lost during the bloody colonization of Mexico. Allow yourself to acknowledge and feel all the emotions that might arise in you. If you have ancestors from the Americas, Africa, or Europe, these stories may live in your ancestral memory. Ancestral trauma is a real phenomenon and can look and feel a lot of different ways. The cellular and emotional memory of ancestral trauma can be present for generations. My

---

* I used "conquest" in quotation marks because words have power. The Spanish tried their best to "conquer" Mexico, and they did indeed destroy codices, libraries, and gardens, and murdered millions of innocent people. However, the spirit of the people, the culture, the ceremonies, and the traditional medicine never have and never will be fully conquered. The fact that so many people are learning about and practicing curanderismo is proof of the people's resistance to colonization.

intention is that some of the practices in this book can become tools for you to support your own ancestral healing.

# We Are Still Here

> When the Spaniards came in, they tried to destroy everything we had constructed. They thought that they had finished us off, but they didn't, because proof of it is the fact that we *are still here*.[1]
>
> —Doña Enriqueta Contreras

In 1519, when Hernán Cortés and hundreds of Spanish soldiers landed on the coast of Veracruz, Mexico, the Nahua civilization was thriving. The Nahua were expert astronomers, agriculturists, architects, poets, mathematicians, artists, midwives, healers, and engineers. Colorful murals decorated the great capital city of Tenochtitlan (site of Mexico City today), which also contained spectacular buildings, fountains, gardens, plazas, and libraries. The Nahua had advanced systems of canals and sanitation, and the Spanish found the city to be immaculately clean, unlike the filthy streets of the European cities they had left behind.[2]

Even Cortés himself was impressed with the great city of Tenochtitlan. In a letter he wrote to the king of Spain, he expressed his concern that nobody would believe him when he wrote of the magnificent civilization he had "discovered":* "It was so wonderful that I do not know how to describe this first glimpse of things never heard of, seen or dreamed of before."

In the following years, the Spanish soldiers, demonstrating an utter lack of humanity, embarked on a calculated rampage that destroyed the magnificent city of Tenochtitlan and decimated the people. Buildings were destroyed, libraries were burned, the wisdom keepers were murdered, and hundreds of thousands of lives were lost.

The tragedy of the invasion of Mexico and its impact on the lives and culture of Indigenous Mexican people are immeasurable. The history of the fall of Tenochtitlan is well documented and is the example I share in this book so that you may have a sense of the scope of what was destroyed. Unfortunately, the

---

\* Of course, the Spanish did not "discover" Mexico, but this is the language the Spanish colonizers used.

Spaniards in their path of destruction brutalized many more Indigenous groups in Mexico and destroyed many other sacred sites, temples, and records of knowledge. Countless Indigenous communities were impacted by colonization, including the Tarahumaras, Maya, Zapotec, Purechepa, Mixtecos, Otomi, Huicholes, and dozens more, and their struggle against colonization continues to this day. Yet, as Doña Enriqueta said, many Indigenous groups have managed to preserve their cultures, traditions, and healing knowledge in spite of the colonizers' attempt to eradicate it.

## Herbal History in Mexico

Mexico has some of the greatest biodiversity in the world. The ecosystems of Mexico include both Pacific and Atlantic coasts, jungles, deserts, plains, valleys, and mountains. In these vast landscapes grow thousands of medicinal plants. Mexico also has rich cultural diversity, in which each cultural group has its own rich and complex history.

It would be impossible to cover all of this history of people and plants in one short chapter. Also, in much of recorded history there has been inherent bias in which stories are valued and which are discarded or deliberately destroyed. When the Spanish invaded Tenochtitlan, they burned libraries and thousands of amoxtli (sacred texts) and destroyed over three thousand medicinal plants.[3] The stories of women, queer and trans people, Black and Indigenous people, and people without money or formal education have often been left out of historical texts as well. Mexican traditional medicine is largely an oral tradition, and much of the history and knowledge has not been written about in books. But that history does exist, and one piece of evidence for it was finally reclaimed in the twentieth century: the Códice/Codex de la Cruz-Badiano.

In colonial Mexico, the Franciscan monks recorded cultural practices of the Indigenous Mexicans in detailed documents called códices/codices.* These codices often included images and were written in Latin, Nahuatl, or both.

In 1536, Franciscan monks established in Mexico City the first college to educate Mexica boys and young men. In 1552, the head of the college commis-

---

* The Nahuatl name for these sacred books is *amoxtli*, which were written on amante paper. Indigenous people in Mexico created thousands of them before the Spanish invasion, but most of them were destroyed by the colonizers.

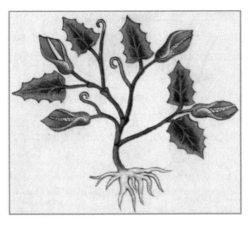

sioned a book to be written as a gift to the Spanish king. This book, *Libellus de medicinalibus indorum herbis*, the *Little Book of Medicinal Herbs of the Indies*, is the oldest surviving written manuscript on Aztec medicine. It became more commonly known as the Códice de la Cruz-Badiano, named after the author, Aztec doctor/healer Martin de la Cruz, who had supposedly converted to Christianity.* Juan Badianus, another Aztec man and alleged Christian convert who taught at the college, translated the text from Nahuatl into Latin.

De la Cruz and Badianus wrote this book under the strict supervision of the Franciscan monks, who watched them closely to make sure nothing was written that could be considered heretical to the Church. In turn, all medical theory of the Aztecs was omitted from the manuscript. Historians have also questioned the authenticity of the book's Aztec herbal knowledge. Much of what was written described herbal protocols that were sometimes more similar to the practices of European herbalism than to those of the Nahua people. I personally wonder whether de la Cruz and Badianus intentionally made up information as a way to resist the theft of their Indigenous knowledge.

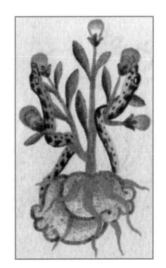

Nonetheless, the Códice de la Cruz-Badiano plays an important role in the history of Indigenous herbal medicine in Mexico. The book documents the use of dozens of different herbs native to Mexico. Each herbal monograph contains a colorful plant illustration, along with a description of its common medicinal use. The book is an invaluable historical

---

* I say "supposedly converted to Christianity" because we really don't know the true spiritual beliefs in the hearts of the authors of this codex. For many Indigenous Mexicans, the choice was to convert to Christianity or be killed. I suspect that, as an act of resistance, many people pretended to be Christians on the surface, but in the privacy of their homes were continuing to practice their Indigenous spirituality.

record of some of the plants most important to the Mexica people, especially since most of their own codices on herbal medicine were burned by the Spanish. It showcases the sophisticated system of taxonomy used by the Mexica people, which was just as developed as European botanists' Linnaean system of Latin binomial nomenclature.

The codex was sent to the royal library of Spain, then eventually stored in the Vatican for four hundred years. It was finally returned to Mexico in 1990, where it now lives in the Museo de Antropología in Mexico City.

Despite this centuries-long effort to bury Indigenous plant knowledge, for five hundred years Mexican people have maintained a strong relationship with medicinal plants. Our plant knowledge endured through oral transmission and also survived in the healing traditions of different Indigenous communities. The practice of plant medicine in Mexico continues to thrive as people maintain relationships with plants as food and medicine and in ceremonies.

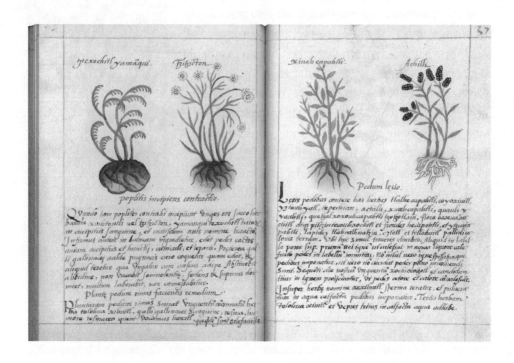

# Brujeria/Witchcraft

The word *witchcraft* has been used for centuries to discredit, demonize, oppress, and persecute traditional healers in Europe, Mexico, and around the world. In Europe during the Middle Ages, as the Catholic Church became a dominant sociopolitical power, anyone who held or practiced different beliefs than those recognized by the Church was accused as a heretic and persecuted. Those considered heretics and accused of witchcraft were often village healers, including herbalists, midwives, seers, and dreamers. People were also drowned, burned, and beheaded for practicing their Indigenous medicine.[4] In Europe between the fifteenth and seventeenth centuries, the Catholic Church executed countless people accused of witchcraft or heresy, of which over 85 percent were women. As traditional healers across Europe were exterminated, there was a very calculated takeover of the practice of medicine by educated males.

How does this relate to curanderismo as practiced in Mexico and in North America today? European colonizers brought with them inherent prejudice against Indigenous healing practices and repeated the same violent acts against Indigenous healers in the Americas as they had witnessed or enacted against their own people in Europe. Soon after the Spanish invasion, Indigenous people in Mexico were also being accused of witchcraft.

As the Catholic Church came to dominate in Mexico, it influenced people's beliefs about their traditional healing practices. Indigenous practices were considered to be the work of the devil and labeled "brujeria." To avoid persecution, many healers adapted and incorporated Catholic beliefs into their work. They began to pray to Catholic saints and incorporated Catholic iconography, such as the crucifix and holy water, into healing rituals.[5]

The persecution of people accused of witchcraft persists, and women continue to be murdered by their accusers.[6] In my interviews with curanderx for this book, several of the elders shared stories of being blamed for practicing witchcraft or of being concerned that their work as curanderx would be negatively associated with brujeria. For some of these elders, the term *bruja* is derogatory. At the same time, however, many younger-generation Latinx are reclaiming the identity of bruja/o/x, and describe themselves as practitioners of brujeria. So today, "bruja" means different things to different people in the Latinx community.

# Three-Headed Serpent

Although today curanderismo may be labeled as "folk medicine," Patrisia Gonzales notes that "it did not stop being Indigenous medicine."[7] Mexican curanderismo is strongly rooted in the healing practices of Indigenous people on both sides of the US-Mexico border, practices that existed for thousands of years before European contact. Over the centuries since colonization, healers from different Indigenous communities were lumped together by dominant colonial powers under the umbrella term *curandero*, and this erasure of indigeneity in curanderismo has continued into today.[8]

Curanderismo evolved from the intersection of people indigenous to Mexico with people from Africa and Europe. As Avila states, curanderismo is the "'three-headed serpent,' the blending together of the people, medicine, and hearts of three cultures."[9] As these three distinct groups of people intermingled, their ideas and practices about spirituality and medicine cross-pollinated. Healers from all three backgrounds exchanged ideas and adopted elements of one another's practices.[10] The healing practices that grew out of this time became a mixture of the traditions, practices, and cosmovision of all three cultures.

In colonial Mexico, the Spanish government passed laws banning anyone who wasn't of European descent from practicing medicine, but many people in rural areas didn't have access to those doctors. This created a space for healers of African and Indigenous descent to step in and serve their communities. However, curanderos also served people from all levels of colonial society, and many Spanish elite sought their services.[11]

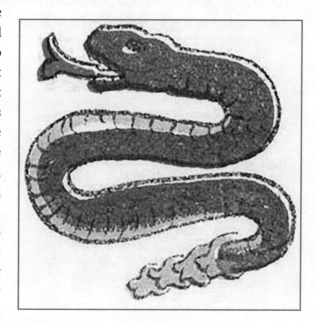

Although these are the three primary roots of curanderismo, each root has its own complex history. The Indigenous people of Mexico and what is now called the southwestern United States have hundreds of different languages, cultures, and healing practices. In the 1500s, Spanish medicine was already a synthesis of different cultural healing systems, including Arabic, Islamic, Greek, and North African medicine. Africans in colonial Mexico came primarily from different regions on the west coast of Africa, where each region had its distinct traditional medicine practices.

# African Roots

Historically, most of the research on traditional medicine in Mexico has focused primarily on its Spanish and Indigenous roots, and the contribution of African people to Mexican curanderismo has largely been ignored.[12] However, African people and traditions have made substantial contributions to the evolution of Mexican curanderismo, and the influence of African, Afro-Latinx, and African American people on curanderismo continues to this day.[13] In colonial Mexico, Afro-Mexican curanderos held significant roles in society, and curanderismo "was one of the ways in which blacks, and especially black women, could gain profit, power and authority in colonial Mexico."[14] Black curanderos were often more sought out than non-Black healers.

African people have been an integral part of Mexican society and culture since colonial times, when enslaved West Africans were forcibly brought to the continent.* Enslaved Africans, most likely from Angola or Congo, traveled with Hernán Cortés when he arrived in Veracruz, Mexico, in 1519. In colonial Mexico, almost a quarter of the population was of African descent; Mexico had one of the largest populations of African people in the Western Hemisphere.[15] By the seventeenth century, Mexico was home to more free Africans than those who were enslaved, making Mexico "home to the most diverse Black population in the Americas."[16] People of African descent outnumbered people of Spanish descent in Mexico until the early nineteenth century, when there was a huge influx of Spanish people settling in Mexico and the Mexican slave trade was abolished.

---

* Some scholars of African history such Ivan Van Sertima document that people from the African continent were present in Mexico long before European colonization.

African people and their traditional healing practices have shaped and influenced Mexican curanderismo in many ways. The popular practice of ventosas, or fire cupping, in which hot glass containers are placed on bare skin to suck out illness and to relieve pain, most likely originated in West Africa.[17] Many plants used today in curanderismo, such ruda and tamarindo, also came from the African continent.

One of the most common practices in curanderismo, la limpia del huevo, the cleansing with an egg, originates from African people and customs. Chickens were imported to Mexico from Europe, and before Spanish contact, Indigenous people in Mexico were not using eggs as a tool to heal sickness and disease. Although many scholars attribute the use of the egg in healing to Spanish origins, in Spain there exist no methods of rubbing an egg across the body for healing and cleansing. However, similar practices of using eggs, feathers, and birds for healings and rituals can be found all across the African continent.[18] Most likely this technique of using an egg for healings was practiced by people of African descent and then eventually adopted by healers of Spanish, Indigenous, or mixed backgrounds.

## Synthesis and Resilience

Indigenous medicine is always adapting to its circumstances.
—Patrisia Gonzales

From its beginnings, curanderismo has been a synthesis of different cultures, which gave birth to a system of healing that contains aspects of each of its cultural roots yet at the same time became something new. This blending of cultural practices can be seen clearly in the use of medicinal plants in curanderismo today. Many of the herbs that are most commonly used in Mexican and Mexican American curanderismo are not plants native to Mexico. Some of these plants, such as manzanilla and romero, came from Europe and have been thoroughly integrated into our traditional medicine. Instead of rejecting the plants of the European colonizers, curanderos who were indigenous to Mexico or Africa found a way to use these plants to support the well-being of their communities.

In the centuries since the Spanish invasion, the practice of curanderismo has been a form of resistance and resilience. Because much of the medical knowledge of the elite levels of pre-conquest society was destroyed, the practice of la medicina tradicional endured as primarily an oral tradition, passed on from one generation to the next. Curanderismo thrived particularly in rural areas and communities that had no access to medical care, where curanderos, playing the role of both doctor and spiritual guide, became the primary source of health care.[19] Most households had someone who knew los remedios to take care of the family, and more expert healers in the community were sought out for more advanced situations. Most often these healers were not actually called curanderos by their community but were referred to as "Esa senora cura," or "El cura susto," or "Ella cura empacho."[20]

Traditional medicine practices have managed to endure for five hundred years as people maintained the knowledge and practices in their homes and communities. Curanderismo continues to be a living, dynamic, adaptable tradition, both in Mexico and in Mexican American communities. Even if an herb is not traditionally used in the Mexican culture, a curanderx may incorporate it into their apothecary. Doña Enriqueta was introduced to reishi, a mushroom used in traditional Chinese medicine, by an acupuncturist, and as she learned about this medicinal mushroom, she was quite impressed with its healing properties. She began to incorporate it into her herbal practice alongside the native and introduced plants and remedies she uses.

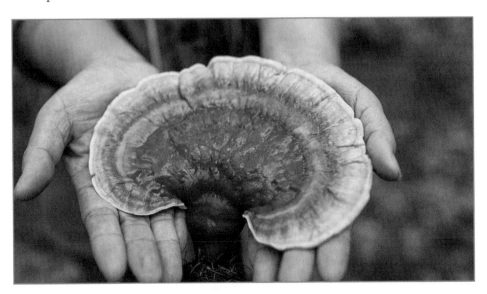

# Curanderismo Flowering in the North

Curanderismo has a rich history in the part of North America now called the United States, especially in the places with large Latinx populations, such as the southwestern states, which had been territories of Mexico until 1848.* During the Mexican Revolution (1910–1920), scores of people fled north, most often settling in California and the Southwest. Throughout the twentieth century, people continued to immigrate to the United States from Mexico and Latin America, often to work as laborers in factories and farms. They formed neighborhoods and communities, where many maintained their cultural practices, including their traditional medicine. On new soil, many planted their beloved crops from Mexico, such as nopal, agave, chili, and maiz, all of which could easily be grown in southwestern gardens. Traditional healers living in the north continued to serve their communities in a similar way as they did back home, as was shared in the story of Trudy Robles.

In the twentieth century, the practice of our traditional medicine in North America was also influenced by the forces of racism, assimilation, and colonization. When Maria Miranda was growing up, her family practiced traditional medicine at home, yet at the same time, she learned from her parents that she should keep certain things secret, for fear of being accused of being a brujo/a. "In the 1950s and 1960s if you had certain abilities, people might think you were a bruja or a brujo. Catholicism did a good job of suppressing. Our people were not free to work with the medicines the way we used to; everything needed to go underground."[21] Eleanor Barron-Druckrey was a student at UC Berkeley in Huchiun in the 1970s and was curious about her Mexican healing traditions. Yet when she tried to learn more from her teachers, she was met with both suspicion and opposition. Even her Mexican American professors labeled it as "superstition" or "brujeria."[22]

In the past few decades, the landscape of curanderismo has shifted and grown. For many generations practiced discreetly in the home or by elders in the community, now curanderismo has flowered into a movement of Latinx people reconnecting to and reclaiming our ancestral medicine. As the consciousness has

---

* The border between the US and Mexico is a social-political construct meant to stop the natural migration of people, to create division, and to criminalize people for crossing. Similarities in practices of traditional medicine can be found on both sides of this "border."

shifted, there is less stigma correlating curanderismo with brujeria, and more proud reclamation of both terms. These seeds of blossoming curanderismo were planted in the political and social movements in Mexico in the 1960s as well as in the Chicano civil rights movement.[23] The Chicano movement inspired Mexican American people to have pride in our cultural roots and resist the pressure to assimilate into Euro-American culture. Many Chicano activists were also working closely with members of the American Indian movement, and more Chicanos began to be curious about their own indigeneity.[24] Chicano cultural and political organizations across the state began to invite Danza maestros and maestras from Mexico to come and help their communities reconnect with their Indigenous ceremonies.[25] In 1968, Angelbertha Cobb (Señora Cobb) held the first Danza Azteca ceremonies in the US in Sacramento/Nisenan territory.[26] In the following decades, organizations that were centered on celebrating Latinx cultural traditions and healing, such Mujeres de Maiz in Los Angeles,[27] began to sprout across the country. Maestros/as, danzantes, and curandero/as from Mexico such as Doña Enriqueta and Estela Román began to travel and teach in North America, and more people from the north started traveling down to Mexico to study with curanderos.

Curandera Elena Avila's groundbreaking book, *Woman Who Glows in the Dark*, was published in 1999, and was the first book about curanderismo to come out in the US written by a practicing Mexican American curandera. The next year, the University of New Mexico, Albuquerque (Tewa Pueblo territory), launched its course on curanderismo, called Traditional Medicine without Borders. Over the years, thousands of students attending the class have had the chance to learn from dozens of Mexican curanderos.

Thanks to these individuals' dedication, a movement dedicated to community healing has grown. Just one example of this is that in 2008, Sol Collective in Sacramento/Nisenan territory began the Curanderismo Class Series, a series of monthly workshops to share the practices of curanderismo to support the health of individuals and communities. Classes were taught by a variety of healers from Northern California and Mexico and were offered by donation to the community. East Bay/Huchiun grassroots women's health collective Curanderas sin Fronteras formed in 2013 and birthed the idea of a mobile healing clinic to serve the Latinx community. The group bought a trailer, stocked it with herbs and supplies, and hit the road to offer its limpias, platicas, and herbal consultations. The same year, the first Healing Clinic Collective (HCC) clinic for women was held in Huchiun/ Oakland. The HCC is committed to "the resurgence of ancestral ways of healing," and community curanderx have always helped organize and offer their services at these clinics. During these clinics, hundreds of people have received limpias, many of whom had never had a limpia before.

# Reflections on the Roots

As I reflect on this history, I can see how my own life path was made possible by the lives of all those who have come before me. When I was first interested in studying curanderismo, it was women who were my elders, such as Trudy Robles and Maria Miranda, who had been active in the Chicano and Danza communities for decades, who supported my work. Unlike so many older than I, I was not accused of witchcraft when I expressed interest in my ancestral medicine. Instead, I was embraced by a community of strong women. Today, curanderx enjoy a time when we can freely study and practice our ancestral medicine without danger of persecution or ostracism. Our ability to practice openly is a blessing, a privilege, and also something not to be taken for granted. We must always remember the struggle and contributions of those who came before us.

The stories in this chapter are only a few threads of the rich tapestry of history that form what we call curanderismo today. Most of the people who tended to this medicine will never be named or recognized. I give thanks to all the known and unknown keepers of this tradition, especially those who preserved the knowledge at risk to their own lives. Tlazohcamati![*] I pray that all of us who walk with this medicine today tend to it in a good way so that it will continue to blossom and be available for many generations to come.

Ometeotl![**]

---

[*] *Tlazohcamati* is commonly translated as "thank you." According to Patricia Chicueyi Coatl, the more accurate translation is "se siente el amor" or "love is felt."

[**] *Ometeotl* is a Nahuatl word that translates to "two sacred energies" or, according to Sergio Magaña, "the union of the heavens and the physical world." It is commonly said at the end of prayers.

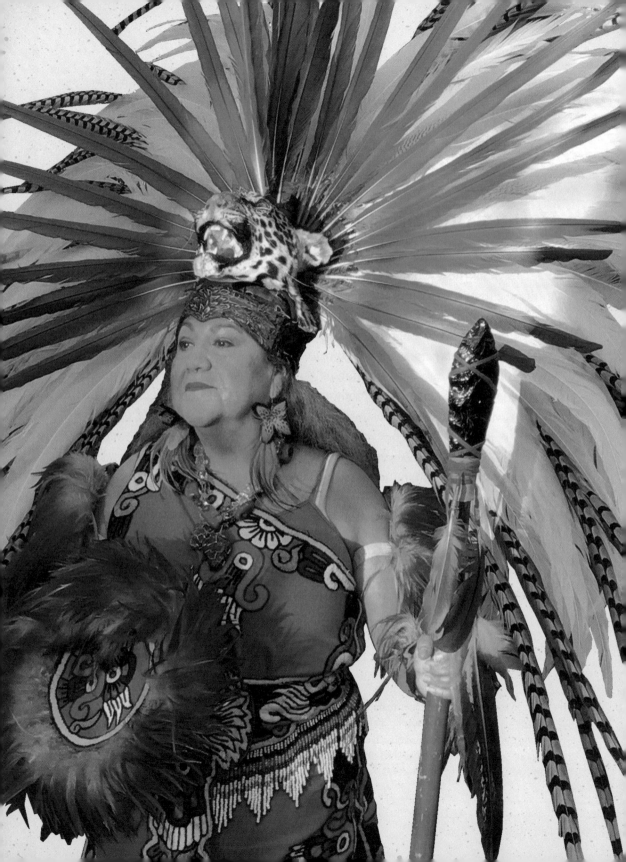

# SPOTLIGHT

# Maria Miranda
## (she/her/ella)

> "Our job as Indigenous people is to help with the times we are living in right now. We need these teachings of curanderismo to help awaken our brothers and sisters: that we are energy beings, we are light beings."

Maria (Chichimeca/Otomi) is the daughter of migrant workers who comes from a long line of medicine women. She is a danzante and capitana of Calpulli Maquilli Tonatiuh, which she has led in Sacramento (Nisenan territory) for over forty years. For decades, her calpulli has hosted annual Danza ceremonias including Dia de los Muertos and Xilonen,* a coming-of-age ceremony for young girls. She has guided countless young women, including her own daughters and granddaughters, through their rites of passage. I had the privilege of meeting Maria through the Sacramento curanderismo community many years ago and consider her to be both a friend and mentor. She is a bright light and a well of wisdom. Every time I speak with her, I leave feeling inspired, cared for, and spiritually nourished.

Maria was born in Texas and "raised with all the remedios in her home; it was natural." When she moved to Oregon in her adolescence, she was confronted with intense racism. Her father, who was involved in the United Farm Workers movement, always taught her to "be proud of who you are." She came to California in the 1960s when, as she remembers, "the whole Chicano movement was in its glory," and became an activist and a member of the Black Berets. Through collaboration with members of the American Indian movement, she began attending meetings at Deganawidah Quetzalcoatl University (DQ-U), the first Indigenous college in California, which was founded in Davis in 1970.

She fondly remembers those days: "I've always been spiritual, but after being introduced to DQ, the little flame inside of me ignited to a bigger flame. I was led

---

* In Nahuatl, *xilonen* means "tender ears of maize."

by Creation and our ancestors. There were medicine people from all around the world. It was our own world there."

She was introduced to the Sacramento Chicano community through members of the Royal Chicano Airforce (RCA)* and began to be involved in Danza Azteca. The RCA had received funding from the city to offer Danza ceremonies for the community. Then the funding ran out. Maria recalled, "A ceremony doesn't stop because it loses funding. I was paying for the ceremonies from my own pocket." She formed her own calpulli, Maquilli Tonatiuh, and was later received as capitana (Danza leader) by a council of elders in Mexico. She was the first Chicana to be recognized this way as a leader in Danza. Maria is a wise, fierce, and compassionate leader who always leads with her heart, who weaves her ancestral medicine into all that she offers the world.

## MARIA MIRANDA SPEAKS:

I was the first Chicana received as a capitana back in the day. I didn't know it back then or know the significance; all I knew is the work had to be done and the ceremonias had to continue.

First and foremost, we must remember we are part of this divine source. With every breath. Creation is living through us, Creation is tasting through us, Creation is touching through us, Creation is reaching out through the medicine we make. It is experiencing everything through us because we are part of Creation.

It is not enough to know, but to know how. This means we need to heal ourselves, to work on ourselves first and practice these ways on ourselves. We need to learn to do our inner work first before we apply it to others.

We are alive right now in these times when the feminine energy was prophesized to return in its full glory. Women have been persecuted; they didn't want us to show our full potential. Now is the time for the women to heal our ancestral damage. We are helping to make the foundation strong again as women. We have been chosen to hold our place again.

That is one of my responsibilities. That is why I was introduced to all these medicine people—it was to help prepare me for what I understand now. We are all the sacred elements. We are the diamond in the rough in the middle of the nahui ollin.**

---

* Sacramento-based Chicano artists and activist collective.

** *Nahui ollin* translates to "four movement" and is the image at the center of the Huey Cuahxicalli, or Aztec Sun Stone (see chapter 10).

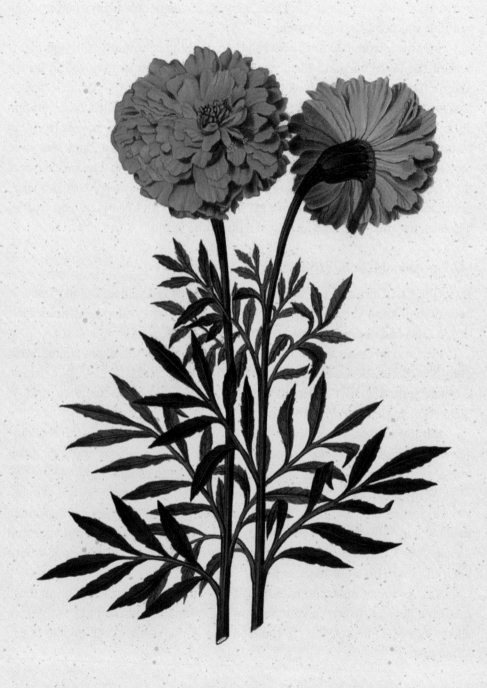

# CHAPTER 3

# Remembering Ancestral Ways of Wellness

I would say that it's a way of life. It's . . . a discipline too, a discipline that you follow because that's how you practice life . . . it's not just a set of practices that you have, but something that you follow in your life that helps you from a basic ailment that you have to a deeper condition of your mind, soul, spirit.[1]

—Estela Román

## The Challenge of Self-Care

An essential part of nuestra medicina has always been the daily practices that people engage in to maintain their health and well-being. Creating conditions for health and healing is not a one-time event but something we must practice each day. Part of self-care is also the maintenance we do to keep our energies clear and flowing.

Without regular self-care, we can slip back into old patterns, and our issues and symptoms may return. One of my intentions for this book is to help you establish daily habits and rituals of self-care for yourself.

I once met with a curandera to address the chronic digestive discomfort I had been experiencing. During our platica, she asked me about my relationships with friends, family, colleagues, and lovers. As I talked about a past relationship, I noticed a tight knot arise in my stomach. The curandera helped me see that whenever I spoke of this person, my stomach clenched and I started to feel angry. She helped me make the connection between my unresolved emotions and the digestive problems I was experiencing.

Next, she gave me a limpia to help me let go of the anger and rage stored in my body. As she sang and prayed, she began to rub the raw egg across my body.

I felt the smooth, cool, firm surface of the egg on my skin and began to burp and fart. I moaned and wept as she swept my body with a bundle of fresh rosemary. As I was enveloped in a sweet-smelling cloud of copal smoke, my body shook as I released old crusty emotions from deep in my bowels. After the limpia, I lay on the massage table feeling exhausted but peaceful. My belly felt soft and relaxed. In the following weeks, I noticed that my digestion had improved, and I could eat normally without pain, discomfort, or gas. I could think of the past relationship without a knot forming in my stomach. I feel grateful for the limpia and the loving expertise of la curandera.

My visit to the healer was just one step in my healing journey. Like a car with a dead battery, I was stalled, and I couldn't easily move out of the situation on my own. Receiving the limpia was like having my battery recharged as the curandera helped reactivate my healing. However, as I was told by the curandera at the end of our session, my work had just begun. She said that I had done an excellent job in releasing some of my aires, but that I must continue to take care of myself in order to maintain my sense of health and well-being. While each of us can be profoundly helped by healers, the most important part of our healing journey is the work we must do with ourselves. This book is intended to be a map to help guide you on this journey of self-healing and self-discovery.

Today many of us struggle to commit to our self-care routines. To commit to our self-care takes a lot of time and energy, and often we feel alone in our efforts. I have seen many of my clients make self-care resolutions, such as to improve their diets, to exercise more, or to quit unhealthy habits like drinking alcohol or smoking. Yet time and time again we all (myself included) slip back into our unhealthy yet familiar habits. When you fall off your self-care path, take a deep breath, forgive yourself, and move on. Celebrate your small achievements. Find people who share your values of healing and wellness, and build community centered on your common understanding. Support one another. Share healthy meals. Take walks together in nature. Garden and make medicine with friends. With our collective focus and intention, we can create a culture that values self-care as our ancestors did.

# Herbal Ally:
## Self-Heal Flower Essence

For those struggling to stay on the path of self-care, one of my favorite allies is self-heal (*Prunella vulgaris*) flower essence, which connects us to our own innate healing wisdom. It helps us know what we need to do to be well and helps us identify the hidden causes of our dis-ease. Self-heal essence is perfect for people starting their healing journey. It strengthens our connection to inner healing guidance, our inner curanderx. I often include it in the very first herbal formula I give to my clients.

Changing our repetitive unhealthy patterns and replacing them with ones that support our well-being are an essential part of healing. Yet this can be hard to do. Self-heal essence helps us make choices that support our health and well-being. When people take self-heal flower essence, they report that making positive change comes with less struggle. They note that their will-power increases and that it is easier to avoid things that are harmful.

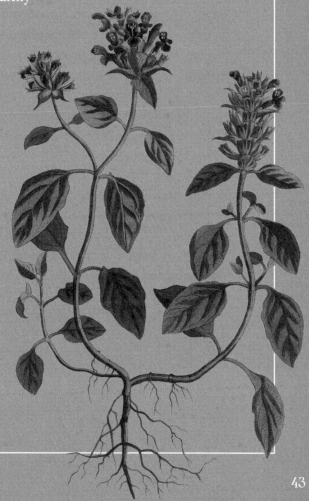

# Care for Community

It is very powerful to remember that we have medicine in our community and can heal ourselves and our families.

—Alejandra Olguin

At some point in human history, all our ancestors knew their place within the sacred tapestry of life. They understood that each individual was part of the sacred whole. They recognized that everything was interconnected: the people, plants, animals, earth, air, and water.

For the Mexica people, this sacred understanding of interrelationship is encoded in the Nahuatl language. Maestra Chicueyi Coatl observes: "From the Nahua people perspective, we are all related to each other, humans with the cosmos, animals, the wind, etc. There's no specific need to have a phrase that highlights this relationship since the whole language and culture highlight this relationship."[2] The Nahuatl language is a binding language and contains words and phrases that convey honor and respect. For example, the suffix *tzin* is commonly added to words as an expression of "venerable essence." *Tonantzin* means venerable Mother Earth, so each time we say "Tonantzin," we are inherently giving our respect to the earth. The concept of honoring all beings is encoded in the whole Nahuatl language. The traditional medicine of the Anahuacan people evolved from this sacred understanding of interrelationship.

Modern medicine rarely makes a connection between individual and community health. We are not encouraged to look out for the well-being of others beyond our immediate family and friends. Instead of participating in a culture of community care, we learn to ignore or stigmatize the people in our communities who are suffering the most, such as people who are poor, houseless, struggling with addiction, or suffering from mental illness. We have forgotten that we are part of the web of life and that our well-being is intricately connected to the well-being not only of other humans but that of all living beings.

# Collaborative Healing

How do we define health in twenty-first-century mainstream American society? In a most simplistic way, health is defined as being free of physical symptoms. For example, when I go to my doctor, she may ask if I am experiencing any symptoms, such as pain, discomfort, or nausea. She may do tests to evaluate the state of my physical body, such as taking my blood pressure or ordering blood work. Yet often the assessment of health is limited to simply the state of my physical body. Although physical health is important, this narrow focus often overlooks the emotional and spiritual needs of the person dealing with the illness.

I believe that many doctors and nurses do care deeply for their patients, but they are restricted by time and the limiting parameters of their professions. When I see a client as an herbalist, I conduct a detailed intake that lasts two hours. I interview my clients about their personal health history and the health of their family. I ask about their childhood, work, relationships, home life, spiritual practice, creative life, and history of trauma. I ask them about their levels of pain, stress, and vital energy. We talk about the quality of their sleep, the foods they eat, their digestion, and even the shape, color, and smell of their bowel movements. In curanderismo we call this platica. *Platica* means talking, and curanderx know that the ability to share one's story and to be listened to with love and compassion is in itself deeply healing.

More people would benefit if curanderx and other holistic and cultural healers worked together with medical professionals for the benefit of the patient. Each practitioner has different strengths and offerings. When someone suffers susto* after a traumatic accident, a physician may help heal the person's broken bones, but a curanderx can help call the person's soul back into their body after experiencing this trauma. When someone receives a diagnosis of cancer, medical doctors offer lifesaving treatments—chemotherapy, radiation, and surgery. Yet a curanderx can give this same person a limpia to release the susto often experienced from receiving cancer diagnosis. By working together, doctors, nurses, therapists, psychiatrists, herbalists, and curanderx can combine their skills and talents to create optimal conditions for individual and community healing.

---

\* Susto is a sudden shock or fright and will be discussed in depth in chapter 11.

# Remembering Ancestral Medicine

> By walking this path and tending to ancestral medicine prac-
> tices, I have been able to deal with some of the most chal-
> lenging of life circumstances (institutional violence, white
> supremacy, etc.) that may have otherwise taken me down.
> Even in the difficult situations, ancestral knowing and light
> still held and guided me.
>
> —Sandra M. Pacheco

We inherit not only the trauma of our ancestors but also their gifts, strengths, and resilience. I believe that one of the best ways to tap into this resilience is to reconnect with our ancestors' medicine ways. For generations, the ancestors of people around the world relied on certain plants for food and medicine. They practiced rituals that supported the well-being of the community. For many, the knowledge of ancestral medicine is still part of their family and culture. For others of us, the healing knowledge in our families and culture has been apparently lost. The forces of immigration, assimilation, colonization, slavery, genocide, and racism have all interrupted the transmission of the culture of healing knowledge in families and communities. However, as my elders have told me, nothing is ever lost. Our ancestral knowledge is still with us; it resides in our bones, our blood, and our DNA.

Everyone, no matter what their history or background may be, has the ability to remember their ancestral medicine. One of my mentors, Hawaiian elder Mr. Hale Makua, said that to "re-member" is to reassemble, to rebuild, to put the scattered pieces of our traditions back together. I experienced this process of re-membering firsthand in my own life when I reconnected with the traditions of my Mexican ancestors. This book, in fact, is the result of all the strands of memory, intuition, dreams, and wisdom from my teachers that I have woven together for the past twenty years on my path of Mexican curanderismo.

# Making Offerings

For those of us who have lost the connection, how can we remember the wisdom of our ancestors? How can we begin to incorporate their healing and life-sustaining practices into our lives today? My elders have taught me that a first step is to make an offering to the ancestors. All cultures have traditional offerings. For example, chocolate, maiz, and copal are common offerings in Mexico. If you don't know your traditional ancestral offerings, you can offer anything that comes from your heart. It can be a prayer, a song, or food. I have been taught to make ancestral offerings outside at the base of a tree because trees symbolically relate to our human family tree. Offerings may also be made at a special place in nature, such as at the ocean or a river, or to a rock; or we can place our offerings on our altars.

When you make your ancestral offering, talk to your ancestors and introduce yourself. It is just like talking to a living loved one, only most of us can't see or hear our ancestors. (Some people who have special powers of perception can see and/or hear spirits.) Tell your ancestors about yourself and what you are seeking from them. Since our ancestors are all at different stages of healing and evolution, I have been advised to call only on well ancestors or ancestors whom you have known and loved while they were alive. Finally, when I make offerings and call on the support of my ancestors, I like to include my plant, animal, and mineral allies as well. For some of my clients and students I have worked with, connecting to their family and ancestors can be difficult and painful. In these situations, I recommend that they start instead by connecting to their ancestral plants. Our relationship to plants does not usually carry the same kind of emotional baggage as our relationship to our families. Yet at the same time, establishing relationship with our ancestral plants or "plantcestors"* can often be the key to remembering our ancestral medicine.

When we are seeking to remember our ancestral medicine, our offerings activate the channels of communication between the spiritual world and us. Once we have made the offering, the next step is to start listening and paying attention to what shows up in our lives. The spiritual world often communicates through intuition, symbols, and synchronicities. Pay attention to your dreams or

---

* Thank you to my friend and colleague Layla Kristy Feghali of River Rose Apothecary, who coined this term.

messages that arise in prayer or meditation. I sometimes receive sudden downloads from my ancestors when I am in the shower. It is helpful to have a journal to write down what you are observing so that you can keep track of the messages.

## ANCESTRAL MEDICINE REMEMBRANCE PRAYER

Beloved Creator
Mother Earth Tonantzin
Ancestors
Please help all people who seek
Remember
Their ancestral medicine ways
So that we may care for our bodies
Hearts
Minds
Spirits
Families
Communities
Animals
Plants
Water
Air
Soil
All life
All beings

As we remember
May we understand and accept
Our sacred responsibility
To our ancestors
To Tonanztin
To future generations
To all beings
Ometeotl!

# SPOTLIGHT

# Marcela Sabin
## (she/her/ella)

> "I had to go on my own path of recovery, to know my own ancestors, to be led back to the original ancestors: the fire, earth, water, and air. They are the ancestors of everyone according to universal law."

Marcela was born in Cordoba, Argentina, of Celtic, Basque, and Saxon ancestry. In 2002, she moved to Huchiun/Oakland to attend graduate school, which is where we met. Marcela has a lifelong interest in working with emotions and trauma informed by an Indigenous perspective. She is the cofounder of the nonprofit Circle of Ancestors, which helps people reconnect to their ancestral traditions. She is also a ceremonial fire keeper in the Ajq'ij community and leads healing workshops for the Latinx community. Marcela has a special sweetness and warmth that make just being in her presence healing.

## MARCELA SABIN SPEAKS:

Each time our writing group met, I lit a small candle. I started to notice that when we gathered around the fire, things were different. I realized in the old days people would gather around the fire; the fire is the core of the kitchen and the home. I asked elders about the fire. One elder told me to look into what my ancestors did. We learned how to make fires from flint. The fires began to be stronger and brought the community together for monthly fire circles.

The fire is a beautiful elder who helps us to transform things. It can be as simple as lighting a candle on your altar or a big fire ceremony. The spirits come through the fire and talk to you in different ways, through the color, shape, rhythm, and sound. Everyone can light a small fire, with natural elements like wood, herbs. It is a good way to get to know the elements around you and to connect with the warmth inside of ourselves.

The limpia is a beautiful tool to work with trauma. We create a container

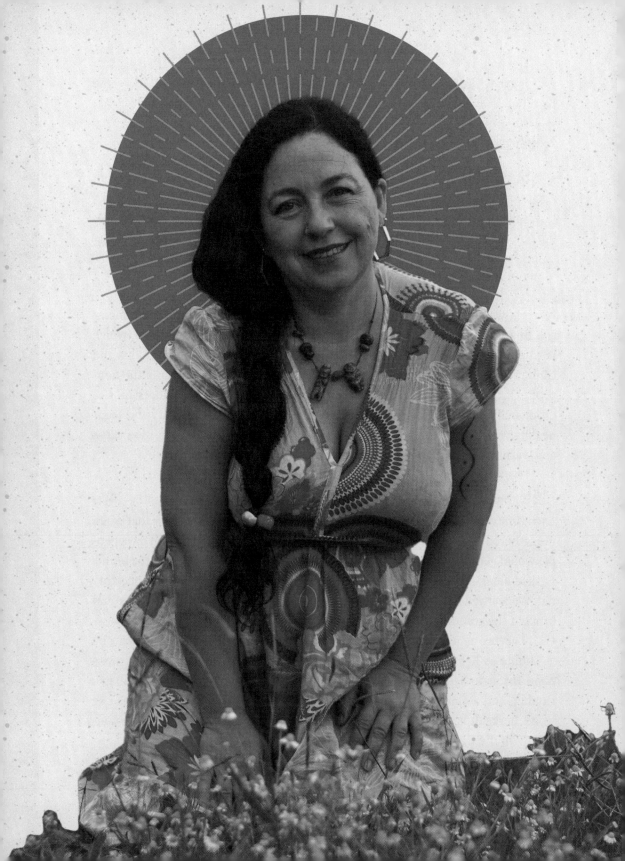

that is based in love, respect, understanding, compassion, and gentleness and based in connection to spirit. This, along with the plants, the copal, and the fire and other elements, creates an opportunity for people to open up and connect. This medicine works in a very safe way with love and makes space for the person to face their aires or their shadow.

In my limpias, I work to create a space for the person to make a connection with those original moments where those aires, those experiences created a trauma. Something got stuck, which may be triggered again with an event in the present. We help people look deeply in themselves, to connect to these moments and release. All the medicine makes this possible.

It's important to work with yourself and to really know who you are, to find what is unique to who you are as a human being. What do you have to offer to others? Why are you here on this planet, in this earth, in this time, and what is unique to yourself now that you are here? This will give you the compass for your life. Find the joy and live the joy and the love. Each person brings something unique, and when we weave all of that together, we become stronger.

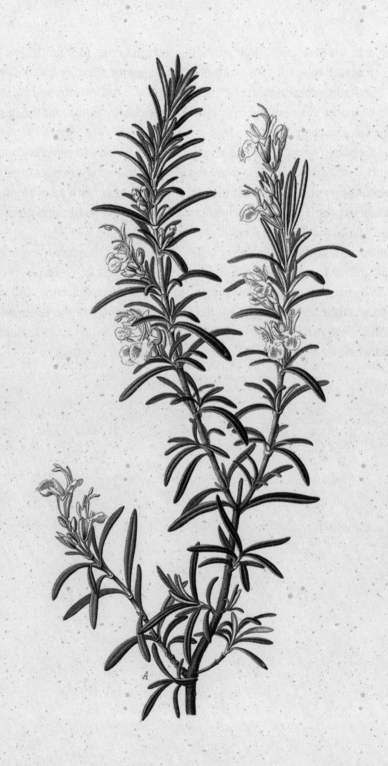

A

# CHAPTER 4

# Self-Care Is a Revolutionary Act

Caring for myself is not self-indulgence. It is self-preservation, and that is an act of political warfare.[1]

—Audre Lorde

The dominant cultural paradigm deliberately ignores the needs of our physical bodies. We are not taught to listen to our bodies. When we are feeling tired or run down, we have not learned to take time to rest. Instead, we drink another cup of coffee or eat something sugary to give us a false sense of energy, and keep on working. Our mainstream culture promotes unhealthy practices, such as overworking, undersleeping, and abusing substances like alcohol, nicotine, and sugar. Many Latinx, Black, and Indigenous communities are food deserts, where people have no access to whole, healthy foods such as fresh fruits and vegetables.

In many communities of color, traditional folk medicine practices like curanderismo have been lost due to the impact of colonization, genocide, and intergenerational trauma. We are taught to fear our own Indigenous and cultural healing practices. We are taught to mistrust herbs and the wisdom of our own bodies.

Each person's health is always a reflection of the health of our society. When poor and marginalized communities are located in toxic environments, individuals are not to blame for their asthma, cancer, or autoimmune disease. Nobody can be expected to know how to eat a healthy diet if the dominant culture is blocking their access to healthy food.

Healing is hard work. Any person who tries to sell you a quick fix for your health problems is either completely out of touch with reality or a con artist. The journey of self-healing requires the strength and fortitude of a warrior. To heal ourselves, we must face our own inner demons, such as the parts of ourselves we dislike or fear. Many of us have suffered from abuse, violence, or other traumas, which take an incredible amount of time and effort to recover from. According to African American trauma therapist Resmaa Menakem, ancestral and intergenerational traumas such as slavery, genocide, and war can remain in our minds and bodies, and they can take generations to fully heal.[2]

To heal ourselves, we must battle the forces of the dominant society that are invested in keeping us sick and disempowered. These include all forces of discrimination and oppression, such as colonization, capitalism, white-bodied supremacy, racism, sexism, ableism, xenophobia, Islamophobia, homophobia, and transphobia. In addition to these toxic forces out in the world, many of us have internalized their messages. It takes determination and willpower to disentangle from these dementors of doom and to protect ourselves from their constant assault.

How do we take care of ourselves when all that we have learned teaches us to ignore or abuse our bodies? An important first step is to not blame ourselves for our poor health. If we had grown up in a culture that valued the well-being of all individuals, many of us wouldn't be suffering from illnesses in the same way.

To heal, we must have the discipline to make changes in our lives. Often, we must let go of familiar habits or addictions that may be contributing to our state of being unwell. Sometimes we are the only one in our family who wants to make healthy changes. Our family members may not understand us; they may judge our new lifestyle choices. We may feel isolated and alone on our healing path.

## Connecting to Our Inner Curanderx

I think every person has a medicine, just like every plant. Everything has purpose. When we are in a rhythm and we are working in a rhythm and we are flowing, there is this magical experience that happens. So I believe everybody carries the medicine.

—Trudy Robles

Our bodies are always speaking to us, sometimes subtly, sometimes dramatically. We may notice a slight shift in our energy and say we are feeling "off" or "not ourselves." The body can also convey louder messages of pain, extreme discomfort, or loss of normal functioning. A common response we have to these messages is often fear. We don't comprehend the language of our bodies, and we often fear what we don't understand. We also may feel afraid because we feel powerless to help ourselves.

Intuition is a vast resource with different functions. Artists tap into their intuition to fuel their creativity. Our gut instinct can alert us when we are in danger. Scientists and philosophers often credit their intuition for their discoveries. Intuition can also be an excellent source of guidance and support for our healing journeys. I call this part of ourselves our inner curanderx.

Our inner curanderx is always communicating to us—we simply need to learn how to listen. A first step is to become aware of how you best tap into your intuitive voice. Sometimes we just need to take the time to be still and listen. Some people receive messages during meditation; others receive guidance in their dreams. The more we practice listening, the easier it becomes. The more we build relationship with our inner curanderx, the more they can guide and support us.

## INNER CURANDERX MEDITATION

To make this more of a ritual, you may choose to start by lighting a candle, sitting at your altar, and blessing yourself with flower water or copal smoke. Take a moment to set your intention. At first, your intention may simply be to connect with your inner curanderx. As you become more familiar with this process, you may have specific questions to ask this part of yourself.

Begin by sitting comfortably on a chair or meditation cushion or by lying down. Choose a quiet space where you can relax.

Close your eyes or lower your gaze and direct your attention inward. Take a few deep belly breaths. Feel the rise and fall of your breath and allow yourself to relax and settle into your body. When you exhale, let go of any stress or distractions. Next, as you inhale, direct your breath to any place in your body that needs attention. If you need emotional support, direct your breath to your heart center in the middle of your chest.

Bring your awareness to your body, tuning into its incredible intelligence.

Feel the wisdom of your cells and your organs, all working together to support your well-being.

Set your intention to connect to your inner curanderx. They are the wise part inside you who can guide and support your healing path. Ask them to appear to you. They may appear as female, male, trans, or gender fluid. They may appear as a person or an ancestor, or may take the form of a plant, stone, light, geometric shape, or magical being. If an image does not appear, you may feel a presence or hear a voice. Notice your physical body. Do you feel this energy living in a particular place?

As you continue to take deep, conscious breaths, tune into this part of yourself. Ask them if they have any messages for you today. If you are working with a particular health issue, you may ask for advice. Take some time to listen.

Do not judge yourself if it is hard to connect with this part of yourself. It can take time and practice. Many of us have not been taught to trust our intuition. For people who are survivors of trauma, going inward may be frightening. Be gentle with yourself.

Before you end your meditation, be sure to thank your inner curanderx for their guidance and support. Sometimes I imagine leaving a gift or offering to show my gratitude.

When you are ready, allow the connection and images to slowly fade. Know that you can continue to return to this part of yourself again and again. Bring your attention back to your breath. When you are ready, slowly open your eyes. Take some time to write down the messages you received.

# Herbal Ally: The Grandmother Plant

The Grandmother Plant (*Tagetes lemmonii*) helps us connect with the wisdom of our abuelas and helps us access the guidance of our inner curanderx. My students have received very direct instructions from this plant, which can be firm but loving and supportive. I recommend working with it in meditations, limpias, or baños, or as a tea, tincture, or flower essence.

# Grounding

> Nature is the highest good in my life. It is Teacher, Mother, Healer, Metaphor, and Home. And Nature is also a set of guiding principles I live by.
>
> —Candice Rose Valenzuela

It can be overwhelming to contemplate the big picture and truly face all the oppressive forces trying to make us sick physically, mentally, emotionally, and spiritually. In addition, we are constantly bombarded with bad news of injustice, hatred, and violence. We are living during a time in human history when climate crisis is a very real threat to our existence as a species. How can we handle this overwhelm?

Each of us has a different default response to stress and overwhelm. Some of us might become angry. Some engage in organizing and political work to fight for change. Others of us might shut down. We may tune out with our favorite addiction or distraction. We binge on alcohol, sugar, or whatever our substance of choice may be. We throw ourselves into work or a relationship.

One of the first and most important steps in practicing la medicina is to learn how to stay centered amid stress and chaos. The forces of patriarchy, white supremacy, colonization, and capitalism want us to be ungrounded. When we are not in our center, we are not in our power and are more vulnerable to harm. How can we learn to stay centered?

Many of us living in urban areas do not have a regular way to connect to Mother Earth Tonantzin, yet this relationship is essential to our well-being and survival. We must practice feeling connected to Tonantzin and engage in activities such as gardening, taking walks in nature, or simply sitting on the earth.

Grounding is also an important practice for curanderx. When we perform ceremonies such as the limpia, our clients may release strong energies. If we are not grounded, we can be overtaken by these energies ourselves. This can be dangerous to us and to our clients. Also, when we learn how to tap into the energy of Tonantzin, we can use this energy to support our healing work.

There are many ways to connect to the earth. Some of the most effective grounding practices require direct contact with the earth, such as

- Walking barefoot on the ground
- Sitting or lying directly on the earth
- Hugging a tree
- Walking mindfully or mediating in nature
- Gardening and getting your hands in the dirt

Sometimes we don't have access to natural spaces or have time to be outside. For those times, I do a simple grounding meditation. I breathe into my belly, feel my body, and imagine I am a tree and feel my roots sink deep into the earth. This helps my energy settle and helps me be more present.

In addition to grounding, another option is to practice feeling the exchange of energy between us and the earth, as described in the meditation that follows. Even though we don't have physical roots, like a plant we are always exchanging energy with Tonantzin. To create more of a ritual, begin by making an offering to Tonantzin. Talk to Tonantzin and ask for support. Tonanztin is a sentient being who listens and responds to our supplications.

## TONANTZIN MEDITATION

To do this exercise, find a quiet place and get into a comfortable position, either sitting, standing, or lying down. Either close your eyes or lower your gaze and bring your attention inward.

Begin by taking a few deep breaths. As you breathe, notice the rise and fall of your breath in your chest and in your belly. Bring your attention to your navel, your ombligo, your center. Our ancestors knew this was a place of power. It may help to put your hands on your belly. As you inhale, imagine that you are gathering any pieces of yourself that are scattered and bringing them back to your body. These scattered pieces may be worries or stresses. Your thoughts may be lingering in the past or jumping into the future. As you inhale, imagine all these pieces of yourself collecting near your ombligo or navel center. As you exhale, let go of anything else that prevents you from feeling present in your own body. Continue to breathe deeply and notice how your energy may have shifted by simply taking a moment to breathe into your belly.*

Once you feel aware of your body and connected to your center, take a few more breaths and begin to feel your connection to Tonantzin. Feel how you are always connected to Tonantzin through gravity. Feel the solidness of your physical body. Feel into the weight of your muscles and bones, which are made from the minerals of the earth. Feel your feet and legs.

Think of your favorite tree. Imagine that you are this tree, with an extensive system of roots. Feel these roots reaching deep into the earth, moving through layers of sand and soil and attaching to something solid like a large stone or another thick root. Breathe into your roots and allow your awareness to sink way down into the ground. Notice how it feels to have roots, how it feels to be planted deeply into the earth.

Just like our plant relatives, we can use our roots to exchange energies with Tonantzin. Feel your roots as conductors of energy. Inhale deeply and feel the earth energy flowing through your roots and into your body. One aspect of Tonantzin, Tlazohteotl, feeds and nourishes us with energy. What kind of energy would you like to call forth into yourself? It may be strength, protection, support, centeredness, or love. Breathe that energy up through your roots and into your body. Send it to all parts of your body, to all your organs and tissues and cells. If there is a place in your body that needs healing, place your hands on that part of your body. Imagine the healing energy from Tonantzin flowing through your hands. If you need emotional support, place your hands on your heart.

Another aspect of Tonantzin, Tlazolteotl, has the ability to accept and transform all of our energetic waste.** Nothing is too noxious; it is all simply energy. With your next exhale, allow yourself to release unwanted energies through your roots into the ground. This may be any emotion, such as fear, anger, stress, or overwhelm. You may release energies that you picked up from other people or from your environment. Ask Tlazolteotl to take these energies and transform

---

* For some people, especially survivors of trauma, learning to connect to your body can be difficult. If this is hard for you, please don't judge yourself or give up. Know that with time and patience you will notice small improvements. If this still feels daunting, I suggest beginning with one of the practices I mentioned earlier, such as walking mindfully in nature or lying with your belly on the earth. These practices help soothe the nervous system and teach you that your body can be a safe place to inhabit.

** For more on these aspects of Tonantzin, see chapter 12.

them. Just as human feces can be transformed into compost for flowers and fruit trees, Tlazolteotl can compost all our emotional and energetic waste. With each exhale, let go of something else and offer it to Tlazolteotl.

Continue to breathe into your roots and feel the exchange of energy between you and Tonantzin. Before you finish, give thanks to Tonantzin. When you feel complete, take a few minutes to bring your awareness back to your breath in your belly. When you are ready, slowly open your eyes and stretch your body. Take a moment to notice how you might feel differently than when you began this exercise. Pay attention to the subtle shifts in your body, emotions, thoughts, or energy field. Take some time to write down your experience and observations.

# Herbal Allies for Grounding

Roots, which grow in the earth, help us to feel rooted. Incorporating root vegetables such as yams, potatoes, parsnips, or beets into our diet can be grounding. An herbal tea made from roots can be both grounding and nourishing.

## NOURISHED AND ROOTED TEA

- 1 part dandelion root
- 1 part burdock root
- ½ part ginger root

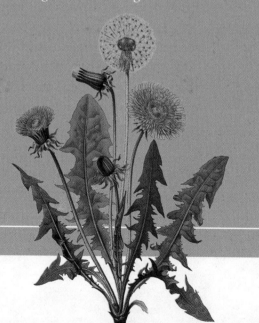

# The Wounded Healer

All that I have learned and have been humbled by in reintegrating nuestra medicina has been through my own process of getting dragged through the underworld! I have come up for air with the help of my hermanx curanderx and maestras, and have willingly gone back into the underworld with their guidance. Curanderismo helps me navigate the place between the shine and the shadow . . . moving like a serpent.

—Angela Raquel Aguilar

To walk the path of a healer, we must constantly work on ourselves. Before we can truly help others, we must first attend to our own wounds. Time and time again I have seen that those of us called to the path of a healer are trained and initiated by undergoing great personal hardships.

Doña Enriqueta suffered many adversities that forged her path as a curandera. At a young age she lost her father. When her mother remarried, she sent seven-year-old Doña Enriqueta off to live with another family. They gave her the chore of tending a herd of goats. As she tended the goats, she was so hungry that she began to eat the wild plants in the mountains. In this way she began to learn about medicinal plants, and as she cared for the goats giving birth, she dedicated herself to becoming a midwife to her human community, too.

Doña Enriqueta lived through many other challenges and tragedies, including the untimely death of her husband, which left her a single mother of five young children. In her platicas with students, Doña Enriqueta often refers to the hardships she has endured, and how much these experiences have taught her. She has told us that one of the most important things she learned is a deep compassion for people who are suffering.

My own personal and family wounds informed my quest to understand the nature of healing and guided my search for ancestral medicine. I grew up in a family with mental illness and addiction on both sides of the family. My maternal grandmother was depressed, agoraphobic, and suicidal. My mother remembers discovering her own mother after a suicidal attempt. My grandmother Hilda died when I was four years old, but her legacy of mental health issues plagues my extended family to this day. In addition, during my adolescence, my father became a compulsive gambler and would be absent for days on gambling binges. His gambling created a lot of stress and instability in our family. I began to struggle with insecurity, shame, and poor body image, and became bulimic. Throwing up offered a kind of release from the stress in my home and family. Today I can understand my desire to vomit as a way to purge myself of my aires, the emotional winds that plagued me, such as fear, anger, shame, and hopelessness. Throwing up was the only way I knew how to release my suffering. This was the only way I knew how to give myself a limpia.

My search to heal myself from my personal and family trauma led me to study acupressure, herbalism, and curanderismo. The best training in supporting others has been the work I have done to heal myself. When I was younger, much of my energy was dedicated to emotional healing from the wounds of my childhood. As an older adult, I have faced more physical health challenges, including diagnoses of an autoimmune disease and cancer. I've observed that we never "arrive" on the path of self-healing. As life unfolds, so do more opportunities to work with ourselves and our medicine.

For people called to be healers, our illnesses, injuries, and traumas can be our greatest teachers. We can allow our wounds to teach us. As we heal, we begin to gather tools and skills to support our own healing, which become parts of our own curanderx toolkit. Eventually these tools we used for our own healing will become the medicina that we share with others.

## Personal Healing Inventory

> If I don't practice my healing for myself, then I am completely disconnected from the Spirit.[3]
>
> —Estela Román

So many factors influence our health. To help myself and my students think deeply about our own healing, I created the Personal Healing Inventory, which contains questions that address many of the factors that I see as influencing a person's state of health and well-being.

Each question will take time and energy to reflect on and write about. You do not need to answer them all at once. Perhaps answer one question a week or work on one per month. Start with the questions that seem most relevant to you in this moment, perhaps the areas of your life that you need to work on the most.

1. PHYSICAL HEALTH

   How would I describe my physical health?
   What foods do I eat regularly, and how does my diet influence my health?
   Do I get enough sleep?
   Do I get regular exercise?
   What is my relationship to alcohol, nicotine, sugar, or other potentially harmful substances?
   What is my overall energy and vitality level?
   What can I do to improve my physical health?

2. EMOTIONAL HEALTH

   How would I describe my emotional health?
   What is my relationship to my emotions?
   Are there certain emotions that tend to dominate me?
   Where do I hold these feelings in my body?
   How do I handle my anger?
   Do I give myself permission to grieve?
   What is my stress level? How do I manage my stress?

3. SPIRITUAL LIFE

   How would I describe my spiritual life?
   Do I have a regular spiritual practice?
   Do I participate in ritual/prayer/ceremony/worship with others?
   Do I have a connection to or a belief in a divine source?
   What are those beliefs, and how are they serving or not serving my health and well-being?
   What are my beliefs about death?

4. CONNECTION TO NATURE

   What is my connection to nature and the sacred elements (earth, air, fire, and water)?
   Do I spend regular time in nature?

Am I connected to the cycles of the moon, sun, and stars?

Do I have relationships with certain plants, trees, rocks, bodies of water, or natural places?

How do I tend to the earth around me?

5. HISTORY OF TRAUMA

What traumas have I experienced in my life?

What support have I received to help me recover?

What areas do I still need to work on?

6. FAMILY AND ANCESTORS

What is my connection to my family, my culture(s), and my ancestors?

What unhealthy family patterns are playing out in my own life?

What healthy patterns have I learned from my family?

What ancestral trauma or patterns of oppressive behavior have I inherited?

What legacy of oppressive/colonial behaviors may be in my ancestral line?

What ancestral gifts have I been given?

7. RELATIONSHIPS

How do I feel about my relationships with my family, friends, partners, community?

Do I feel safe and supported in my relationships?

How do my relationships impact my overall health?

How do I give and receive support?

Am I able to forgive people in my life who have hurt me? How do I participate in community?

8. HOME LIFE

How do I feel about my home life?

Is my living space supporting my health and well-being, or is it a source of stress?

What environmental toxins might I be exposed to where I am living?

9. WORK/SCHOOL/VOCATION

How much do I enjoy my work (or school)?

How does my relationship to work affect my health (working too much, unemployment, underpaid, toxic work environment, etc.)?

How is my work/life balance?

10. CREATIVITY, REST, PLAY, AND PLEASURE

How much time in my life do I have for creativity? Rest? Play?

What do I do regularly for rest and relaxation?

How do I nurture my creativity?

What gives me pleasure?

How much time do I allow myself to engage in what gives me pleasure?

What recharges and reenergizes me?

11. IMPACT OF OPPRESSION AND/OR PRIVILEGE

How has my health been influenced by oppressive societal factors such as colonization, racism, sexism, classism, homophobia, transphobia, ableism, Islamophobia, or xenophobia?

What are things I can do for myself to support my resilience?

What privilege do I have based on my race, class, gender, and so on?

How am I working to address these in my life?

12. SELF-CARE AND COMMUNITY CARE

What do I do regularly for self-care?

How can I improve my self-care to support my healing intentions?

How can I support others in my life to better take care of themselves?

How can I contribute to the health of my community?

13. HEALING INTENTIONS

What are my healing intentions for myself?

What are my self-healing goals?

What are my goals for the next month? For the next four months? For the next year?

As Maestra Maria Miranda says, "Where intention goes, energy flows." As you set your intentions, your life will naturally navigate toward those goals. Writing down your intentions brings more energy toward their manifestation. Place your written intentions somewhere in your home where you can see them daily. As you read these intentions often, they will germinate like seeds in your unconscious.

## SPOTLIGHT

# Candice Rose Valenzuela
## (she/her/they/them)

> "A wild seed, a seed that blows on the wind and seeds itself into new territory. That's me. It wasn't specially picked, sprouted, nurtured, and pruned. It was sown on the wind by birds and came into being through the forces of nature."

Candice identifies as a multiracial/multiethnic Black person who was born and raised in Watts, California, to an African American mother and a Mexican father of mixed Indigenous and European descent. Candice is a parent, teacher, trainer, and trauma-informed yoga and mindfulness instructor, and is currently training to be a therapist. I first met her when she became my student. She is a bright light, brilliant thinker, and writer, and I feel blessed that our paths have crossed.

### CANDICE ROSE VALENZUELA SPEAKS:

The immediate family who raised me was Christian and very adamant about their faith. We were taught that Indigenous ancestral ways were demonic and bad. I was taught to fear anything spiritual, which actually increased my interest in alternative spirituality, healing, and the occult. At the age of sixteen, I rebelled and refused to attend church anymore.

Later, in college, I was researching "Africanisms": African customs, ways of speaking, thinking, and being that persisted through the generations of African enslavement in the US. I found several ancestral practices still present in my family, though their meanings had been lost over the years. For example, I was taught to never sweep someone's feet, and if you do, to spit on the broom, a custom that has its roots in the spirituality of enslaved Africans. I was proud to find these ancestral memories still surviving right under our noses despite colonization and oppression.

It felt essential to my own personal healing and development to connect to my ancestral roots. I was inspired by the sincretismo that was present in Santería,

and that led me to also look at other syncretic practices such as curanderismo. These traditions arise out of adaptation, survival, and the solidarity that arose between colonized cultures for resistance and survival (just like me). Santería and curanderismo both contain African, Indigenous, and colonizer roots, just like me.

Most of my life, I did not feel visible or valued in my body and the lineages it carries. Finding these spiritual paths was very affirming, like a homecoming to me, to find a place where I am seen, valued, and where I can belong. I no longer felt pulled to identify as "part this" or "part that," as a multiethnic person, but rather as a whole lineage, a whole person, a whole legacy of survivals that began long before me and long before colonization.

I use ancestral teachings when I am caring for my child (they/them). I teach them how to connect with plants, plants' roles in our lives, and how to love them. I foster their relationship with nature, as being just as important as their relationship with me or any other person.

When I work with clients, I take time beforehand to center in my own ancestors' guidance and protection through prayers, smoke, and intentions. I also pray for the ancestors of my clients—whether individuals or communities. I ask that all good ancestors be with us in our work, and that our work together promotes healing seven generations forward and back. If I am visiting a community or client in person, I arrive early and make prayers to the land, spirits, and plants that guard and care for that place. I ask permission to do the work with my client(s), and I ask for spiritual support.

In addition to my therapeutic skills, my ancestral and spiritual awareness is always with me, helping me to hold the container. I've found this ancestral perspective in counseling to be particularly helpful and healing for QTPOC and BIPOC clients, by allowing them to touch into a deeper recognition and awareness of who they are beyond dominant paradigms.

Ancestral medicine is the primary way that I take care of myself in this work, and to maintain the integrity and confidence I need to support people and communities through very difficult circumstances.

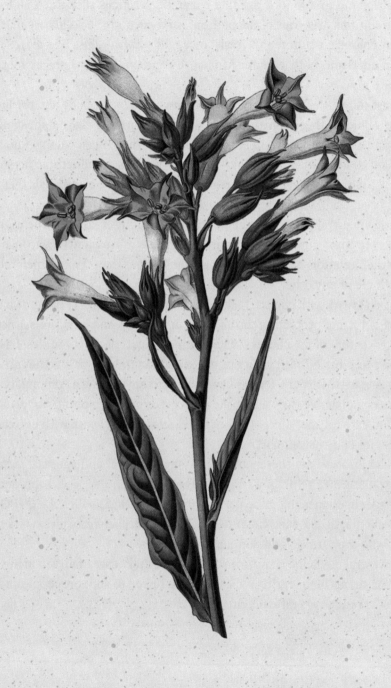

# CHAPTER 5

# Creating Sacred Space

Prayer is the foundation of the work of a curanderx. We pray, sing, and make offerings to plants when we plant our herbs and before we harvest them. We pray as we make our teas, prepare our baños, or process our herbs for tincture. We pray with and for the people who seek out our services. Each part of our work is a prayer in action for the healing of our families, our communities, and the world. Prayer is one of the elements we call on to create sacred space. There are infinite ways to create sacred spaces, and each curanderx has their unique way of doing it. One common thread for most of us is that it requires working with the forces of the universe and nature. We learn to build reciprocal relationships with the sacred energies that we work with, so that we are not just taking from them but also learning how to give back.

## Stepping out of Ego-Driven Healing

As healers, we feel good being able to help people! But we have to be aware of whether our acts of helping are genuinely for others or to give ourselves a boost. Often as healers, we learn to value ourselves by the measure of how much we do and how much we help. As a young woman struggling with my mixed-race identity, I found that people would be more likely to accept me when I was helping them. So, early on, my desire to be a healer was wrapped up in my self-esteem and the sense of importance I felt when I helped people. And I felt good about myself because I had "done" something helpful.

Then, as I spent more time around traditional healers, I learned that their perception of their work differs from a modern ego-based paradigm. Traditional healers are motivated not by a sense of personal importance or superiority but often by a strong desire to help their community. Moreover, time and time again I heard curandero/as say that they were not the ones "doing" the healing. Instead, they talked about calling forth the healing forces of the universe to assist their work. They view the ultimate healer to be a divine force that may be called by many names, such as Dios/a, Jesus, La Virgen de Guadalupe, or Espiritu Santo. These curandero/as possess a deep reverence for the divine forces that they see as responsible for the healing, and they see themselves as being in service to this divine power. To be in service to the divine instills a sense of both respect and humility, as it comes with an understanding that to have the honor of working with these energies is a gift. To continue to access this gift, the healer must maintain right relationship with the sacred energies, which requires both responsibility and commitment. This commitment is woven into the daily life of each healer. For example, Maestra Estela regularly enters the temescal to pray and take care of herself. Doña Enriqueta tends to her healing altar with daily offerings of fresh flowers and keeps her healing space immaculately clean.

To transition from being an ego-based healer is a major paradigm shift for those of us trained in a colonized world. For myself, it is an ongoing process to keep my ego in check. I often ask myself, What is motivating my work? What am I getting out of this? Am I doing this to gain prestige and recognition? Am I posting about my work on Instagram so that I get more followers? Or I am motivated by a genuine desire to be of service and help my community?

As I have shifted from the belief that I am "doing" the healing work, the first step for me has been to consciously invite sacred energies, energías sagradas, to participate in the healing session. Whether I am doing a limpia, talking with a client, or making medicine, I always start by welcoming the divine energies. What are these divine energies? For each of us doing healing work they will be different, depending on our particular cultural background and spiritual beliefs. In my work, I always invite in the energy of the Creator and of the earth, Tonantzin. Other healers may invoke La Virgen de Guadalupe, Mayahuel, or Oshun. In addition to invoking these energies, each healer learns to call in their own ancestors, spirit guides, and herbal allies. I like to welcome my ancestors who were herbalists, curanderas, and healers from all of my bloodlines. I also call in my beloved mentors who have passed, my father, and the spirit of some of my favorite plant allies such as tobacco and yarrow.

As we consciously engage with energies beyond ourselves in our work, we start to shift from the ego-based perspective that we are the ones doing the healing. We recognize that our healing work ultimately requires collaboration with many sacred energies and elements. I ask myself: What sacred relationships must

I maintain to do my work? What is my responsibility to the earth, the elements, the plants, the ancestors, and all beings who support my work as a healer?

# Aligning with the Energies of the Cosmos

As danzantes we move energy, we work with the four sacred elements. Each and every one of us is part of creation as we are a ripple in it, and when we move and dance, we are moving energy and we are contributing to the whole.

—Maria Miranda

One aspect of healing work that is common for traditional healers across the world is aligning with the elemental energies of the earth. Our ancestors were connected in a daily way to earth, fire, air, and water. They tended to the earth and cultivated corn, beans, and squash. They tended hearth fires to cook their food. They made offerings at sacred springs and held ceremonies to honor the rain. From their daily lived experience, they observed the different qualities of each element. Our ancestors also observed the cycles of the earth, the sun, the moon, the stars, and the planets and understood their relationship as human beings to the energies of the cosmos.

As healers who are remembering our ancestral medicine ways, we must take the important step of learning how to be in relationship with the energy of the elements. There are many ways to do this. We may learn about water by taking ritual baths or by swimming in a lake, ocean, or river. We may learn about fire by lighting a candle or tending to a ceremonial fire. We may learn about earth by tending to our gardens or simply spending quiet time in nature. We may learn about air by working with the sacred smoke in our popoxcomitl or by using our voice for poetry and song.

Another step to remembering our ancestral medicine ways is to learn how to work with the energies of the cosmos. These cosmic energies include the power of the four cardinal directions (east, west, north, and south), the heavens (the sun, moon, stars, planets, comets, and so on), and Tonantzin. The practices to align with these cosmic energies vary among different curanderx. For me, participating in Danza Mexica was an important doorway that grounded me in an ancestral ceremonial cosmovision that in turn influenced the way I create a sacred container for my healing work.

# Danza Mexica

> Danza gives us, Indigenous people, the opportunity to practice our ancient traditions and a way to rediscover the conocimiento or knowledge our ancestors inherited to us and is also a way for us to honor them.
>
> —Patricia Chicueyi Coatl

When I first started to study curanderismo in the early 2000s, I didn't know many other people who shared my interest. I felt lonely, and longed for companions on the path. When Estela Román taught her first workshop in Sacramento/Nisenan territory, I connected immediately with the small circle of women who had organized the workshop. I was so grateful to find like-minded spirits who, like me, were passionate about reconnecting with ancestral medicine. Two of these women were Trudy Robles and Maria Miranda, both of whom were very involved in the ceremonial community of Danza Mexica. Maria Miranda was the founder and capitana (leader) of Calpulli Maquilli Tonatiuh, and Trudy was the lead sahumadora, or keeper of the sacred fire. Maria and Trudy warmly welcomed me and my partner into their community and introduced me to the world of Danza Mexica. Danza allowed me to connect to the living cosmology of my ancestors, and taught me to dance and sweat my prayers.

Danza Mexica is a ceremonial practice originating from different cultural groups in Mexico, including the Mexica, Chichimeca, Teotiuacan, and Olmec.[1] For generations, the tradition of Danza has been kept alive in spite of the colonizers' violent attempts to eradicate it.* The tradition of Danza has grown and

---

* After the invasion of Mexico, the Spanish colonizers viewed all Indigenous practices as "savage" and "the work of the devil," including Danza. Danzantes caught practicing their ceremonies risked persecution or death. In 1520, in a bloody rampage known as the Massacre at the Temple of Tenochtitlan, Spanish soldiers invaded a ceremony at Tenochtitlan in honor of Huitzilopochtli, committed unspeakable acts of violence, and murdered the danzantes. I mourn, rage, and pray for these lives lost. That Danza continues to flourish today is a testimony to the strength of the tradition and the resilience of the people.

spread throughout Mexico, Turtle Island, and the world. Today Danza is both a cultural movement and a political act of resistance to colonization.* According to danzante and scholar Jennie Marie Luna, "Since the arrival of Europeans, Danza has served as a tactic to counteract cultural and spiritual genocide."[2]

All of the elements of Danza resonated deep in my bones: pungent wafts of copal smoke, ornate regalia, billowing feathers, colorful altars of flowers, bundles of rosemary, the resonant call of the conch, and the collective rhythm of our movement. After entering the world of Danza, I found a grupo closer to home, Calpulli Huey Papalotl, based in Huchiun Ohlone territory (Berkeley, California) and led by Maestra Chicueyi Coatl, danzante and Anahuacan scholar. Through her teachings on the Anahuacan cosmovision, I learned about Nauhcampa, the sacred energies of the four directions, and have been able to apply this knowledge to the way I create sacred space in my healing work.

# The Secrets of Curanderismo

Back in 2011, Jefa Maria Miranda was one of the very first guest teachers in the Curanderx Toolkit class. In class she taught us about the connection between curanderismo and Danza. I remember her saying something that has been forever etched in my memory: "The secrets of curanderismo are hidden in Danza." Her words intrigued me and inspired me to learn more. Years later I am still uncovering the meaning of Maria's words, and I will most likely be reflecting on them for the rest of my life.

One connection between Danza and curanderismo is in the role of the sahumadorx, who tend to ceremonial fire and smoke and also hold a lot of responsibility within the calpulli. In many ways, the training of a sahumadorx is like the training of a curanderx. According to Chicueyi Coatl, sahumadorx are trained to care for the momoxtli (altar) and tend to the four sacred elements.[3] Before each ceremonia, the sahumadorx help create the momoxtli, which is often elaborately designed and constructed from materials such as flowers, maize, plants,

---

* The history of Danza is complex and multilayered. I am not a historian, but I think it is important in the context of this book to share some history of Danza. For more history, as well as a contemporary analysis of the Danza movement, I highly recommend Jennie Marie Luna's dissertation *Danza Mexica: Indigenous Identity, Spirituality, Activism and Performance*, found in the endnotes.

and colored sand. Sahumadorx learn to carry the sacred fire (popoxcomitl) and are taught how to work with the smoke (air) for prayer, healing, and protection. During the Danza, sahumadorx weave throughout the circle of danzantes offering copal smoke, staying alert, and making sure everyone is safe. They learn how to protect the circle of danzantes from potentially harmful energies, such as threatening people from outside the sacred circle, or from any danzante within the circle whose energy may be disruptive. Sahumadorx are also trained to support other situations that may arise, such as if a danzante passes out from dehydration or seems to be overtaken by a spiritual entity. Sahumadorx also use herbs to administer first aid to weary and injured danzantes in ceremonias. During ceremonias, sahumadorx work tirelessly and are often the first ones to arrive and the last ones to leave. Fulfilling each responsibility of a sahumadorx is also training to be a curanderx: creating sacred space, building altars, supporting ceremonies, protecting the community, healing, administering first aid, offering spiritual support, and intervening in times of emergency.

Another similarity between the path of a danzante and that of a curanderx is that neither role is a casual pastime, but instead a calling, a lifestyle, and a spiritual commitment. Both require dedication and much personal sacrifice, strength, perseverance, and humility. Luna writes, "Danza Mexica, in its origins, was a spiritual practice, a way of life and a way to connect the mind and body to the universe."[4] Danza gave me not only the gift of learning my ancestral cosmovision but also the opportunity to experience this cosmovision as an embodied physical practice. We do not simply intellectualize the cosmovision but learn to move our bodies in alignment with the sacred movement and mathematics of the cosmos. We dance around the circle and greet each of the sacred directions. We shake our sonajas (rattles) with arms outstretched and offer our prayers to the east, west, north, and south, to the cosmos and the earth. We breathe in the aroma of copal smoke and feel the reverberation of the conch shell resonate in our bones. Our bodies spin like planets rotating around the sun. Our feet move swiftly to the voices of our ancestors speaking through the huehuetl (drum). With arms outstretched, we salute the sacred energias of the cosmos.

# Anahuacan Cosmovision:
# The Universe as a Flower

In the Anahuacan cosmovision, the universe is a flower. This cosmic flower has three distinct but interconnected worlds: the four cardinal points of the earth, the thirteen heavens, and the nine underworlds. The earthly realm is called Tlaltícpac, translated as "the place where we live," and forms the flower's four petals.[5] Each petal represents one of the four cardinal directions: east, west, north, and south.

Above Tlaltícpac are the thirteen heavens, or Ilhuicatl, which are represented by the pistils of the flower. Distinct sacred energies dwell in each heaven, and each has a different purpose and function. Below Tlaltícpac exists Mictlan, the realm of the nine underworlds, which correspond to the stem of the flower. These underworlds represent the places where one's spirit must travel after dying and losing the physical form, and also relate to the places that we travel in the dream state.

This cosmovision is complex and multidimensional. The four earthly realms, thirteen heavens, and nine underworlds of this cosmic flower relate to the order of creation in the universe. This cosmovision also corresponds to the path of human evolution and spiritual development. Encoded in this cosmology is the understanding that everything within the universe is also reflected within human beings. Every heaven, each underworld, each part of the flower is related to phenomena in the universe and also within our own body and psyche.

# Nauhcampa

Although human beings across the globe have countless differences, one thing that we all share is the experience of living on planet earth. No matter where we live, we all share the same earth, sun, moon, and stars. On every continent on earth, the sun rises in the east and sets in the west. From this collective experience of our place in the cosmos comes a universal understanding of the four directions. In the Anahuacan cosmovision, the four directions (which relate to the four petals of the flower) are called Nauhcampa. Nauhcampa can be translated as "los cuatro rumbos" or "four directions of the winds." *Nahui* corresponds to the number four, but it has a more complex meaning. Nahui comes from two Nahuatl words, *nantli* (mother) and *hui* (order). A broader translation is "the order of the mother," or the order of Mother Earth Tonantzin.[6] Here on earth we have four seasons, four phases of the moon, four phases of the day, and Nauhcampa, the four directions.

The energies of Nauhcampa represent forces both inside and outside us. Each direction has its own unique properties and gifts, which we can cultivate within ourselves to use for healing, transformation, and spiritual development. When we work with the different energy of each of the four directions, we bring particular qualities to our healing work.

## Tlahuiztlampa (*Rumbo Este, East Direction*)

**Tlahuiztlampa** translates to "place of the light"; it corresponds to the east direction. As the direction of the rising sun, the east relates to new beginnings and the start of a new cycle. Tlahuiztlampa is sometimes referred to as the place of "masculine" energy, but this energy is not limited to people who identify as male. All beings, regardless of gender, possess qualities of masculine energy. Quetzalcoatl, the legendary feathered serpent, is one of the sacred energies of this direction. Quetzalcoatl relates to the energy of wisdom and enlightenment and is associated with the planet Venus as the morning star. Xochiquetzal (flowering quetzal), the energy of creating beauty and harmony on earth, also corresponds to this direction. Tlahuiztlampa corresponds to the fire element, the number thirteen, and the colors white and yellow.

### CONNECTING TO TLAHUIZTLAMPA

A simple way to invite the energy of Tlahuiztlampa into your healing session is to build your altar in the east or simply to face the east direction to pray. Include feathers or white or yellow items or candles on your altar. The energy of Xochiquetzal inspires beauty, so we can connect with its energy through all forms of artistic expression.

To connect with Tlahuiztlampa, go outside in the early morning to observe the sunrise. Many spiritual traditions consider early morning to be a potent time for spiritual practice, and the early morning rays of the sun have many beneficial effects on your body. Sunrise is a good time to meditate, stretch, pray, or sing.

As the sunrise brings a sense of freshness and light, I have found its energy to be helpful for working with depression, sadness, and grief. Because the east is associated with Quetzalcoatl and wisdom and enlightenment, it is also a good direction to work with when you need guidance about something in your life.

A very simple practice is to go outside during sunrise, face the eastern horizon, and take 13 (or 26, 39, or 52) deep and conscious breaths. Breathe in the energy of the new day and the light of the morning sun.

## GRIEF HEALING PRACTICE

Sunrise is a very special time of day to connect with the energy of renewal and rebirth. Each sunrise, we have the opportunity to greet the sun and begin a new day. Sunrise brings hope and light to us when we feel sad, depressed, or full of despair.

To support yourself when you are sad, grieving, or depressed, wake up early and observe the sunrise. Go outside to greet the sun and allow the colors and light of the dawn sky to wash over you. Listen to the songs of the birds. Make an offering to the sun, Tonatiuh, introduce yourself,* and ask it to support your healing. Feel the light of the sun on your face and invite its light into your heart. Pay attention to how you feel and how this sunrise medicine helps lift your heavy heart. To maximize the effects of this practice, try doing it for four or thirteen days in a row.

## Cihuatlampa (Rumbo Oeste, West Direction)

**Cihuatlampa** translates to "the place of the feminine energy" and corresponds to the west direction and to the time of sunset. Cihuatlampa is ruled by the energy of Xipe Totec, the Lord/Lady of Shedding, a deity associated with springtime, new vegetation, renewal, and healing. The Cihuateteo (translated as "female deities") also live in the west. The Cihuateteo were women who had died in childbirth and

---

* Maestro Hugo Nahui teaches that we must always introduce ourselves to the sacred energies. Say your name out loud to them, and eventually the energies will recognize you by the vibration of your name.

were thus considered to be warriors.* Each day the Cihuateteo guide Tonantiuh across the sky from its zenith (high noon) until the sun's "death" at sunset.[7]

The west is the direction where the sun sets. Cihuatlampa relates to the end of a cycle and the energy of letting go, renewal, and regeneration. It corresponds to the number seven, the element of earth, and the color red.

Cihuatlampa helps us tap into the divine feminine energy that is inside all of us, no matter what our gender or gender identity. As the direction of the Cihuateteo woman warriors, Cihuatlampa can empower all who identify as women. Cihuatlampa can also support those who identify as male or who are trans, nonbinary, or gender fluid in connecting with their own feminine energy.

## CONNECTING TO CIHUATLAMPA

Cihuatlampa energy helps us let go of things that no longer serve us, and working with it can be helpful for rituals that mark transitions of any kind. To bring the energy of Cihuatlampa into your healing, build your altar in the west or conduct your ritual facing in the west direction. You may also hold your ceremony during the time of sunset or include red candles and items on your altar.

A simple practice to harness the energy of Cihuatlampa is to go outside during sunset, face west, and observe the sunset. As you meditate on the setting sun, allow the red, orange, and pink colors of the sky to wash over you. Like those of sunrise, the colors of light during sunset have many healing benefits. By observing the colors of light at this time of day, our bodies are prepared to unwind, rest, and sleep.

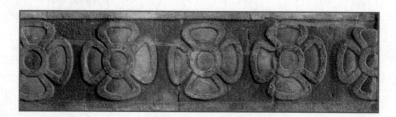

---

\* According to written history, the Cihuateteo are malicious spirits who cause harm, illness, and death and also prey on children. However, according to oral tradition, the Cihuateteo are actually beneficial spirits who seek to give love and aid to human beings. Sergio Magaña teaches that because the Cihuateteo never had the chance to fulfill their dream of being a mother, they are hoping to fulfill their lost dream by giving their mothering to living human beings who seek their support.

# Ceremony at the Hole

Once during a curanderismo retreat, Maestra Estela Román conducted a group ceremony in which we worked with the energies of Cihuatlampa. Thirteen people were participating in this summer retreat, which was held on a friend's land in Northern California/Pomo territory. About an hour before sunset, Estela guided us outside to a small grove of pine trees where we had a clear view of the sunset over the rolling foothills.

We began our ceremony by greeting each direction with prayer and music. As we moved to face each direction, we reached our arms up to welcome the energias. One woman played a soft heartbeat on her drum, and another blew the conch. Some women shook their rattles/sonajas, and others offered pungent copal smoke from their popoxcomitl.

After opening the circle, we made an offering to Tonantzin and asked permission to work with her. Next we dug a hole about two feet deep in the west direction. One by one, each person stepped up to the hole so that they were facing west and the sunset. Estela's intention was for each of us to use our time at the hole to release and let go. The rest of us stood behind the person in a half-moon shape so that we all were facing west. We sang, prayed, played instruments, and burned copal to support each person's healing.

As the healing ceremony began, one by one people took their turn to kneel down at the hole to release. As people let go, they cried, screamed, and shook. The rest of us supported each person with songs and prayers. The ceremony lasted for hours, and by the end of the ceremony there were only a few of us remaining. We smudged the hole, thanked the energies, and filled the hole up with dirt.

# LETTING-GO RITUAL

As it relates to the end of the sun's cycle each day, or the "death" of the sun, Cihuatlampa is a perfect energy to connect to when we need to let go of things that no longer serve us, including emotions, situations, jobs, relationships, past traumas, or behaviors and addictions. The energy of Cihuatlampa can be also be helpful for rituals that mark transitions of any kind, including moving, ending a relationship, starting a new job, or losing a loved one. We can work with Cihuatlampa to honor all life passages, including graduation, getting married, or going through puberty or menopause.

The best time to hold rituals for letting go is at sunset, the special time of day when the world transitions from day to night. Find a place outdoors where you can sit quietly and watch the sunset. Pay attention to your breathing as you meditate on the sunset. The number that corresponds to this direction is seven, so try taking 7 (or 14, 21, or 28) deep and conscious breaths and inhale the energy of the setting sun. As you exhale, imagine what you want to let go of in your life, and release those things through your breath as an offering to the west direction.

You may decide to build a small altar for yourself in the west direction. Make an offering to Cihuatlampa and ask for assistance in letting go. You may choose to say out loud what you are letting go, or you may choose to dig a small hole and bury items that represent what you want to release, or simply write words on a piece of paper to bury. If you dig a hole, first make an offering to Tonantzin and ask her permission.

Cihuatlampa corresponds to Xipe Totec, the renewal of corn and the energy of regeneration. In your letting-go ceremony, you also may ask for renewal in your life. Letting go is an essential part of ushering in new life. We can observe this pattern in nature. A tree will lose its leaves in the fall and move through a period of dormancy until new green buds sprout in the spring. When we let go of something in our lives, we are making room for something new to sprout and grow. To amplify the energy, repeat your ceremony for four, seven, fourteen, or twenty-eight days.

# Mictlampa (Rumbo Norte, North Direction)

**Mictlampa**, the north direction, means "place of the dead" and relates to our ancestors and all who have died. Mictlampa also corresponds to dreams and the unconscious mind. The element of wind, the number nine, the moon, and the hour of midnight are all associated with Mictlampa.

Mictlampa is ruled by Tezcatlipoca, the lord of the underworld. The name Tezcatlipoca is formed from two Nahuatl words: *tezcatl*, which means mirror, and *poca*, which means smoke. Tezcatlipoca can be translated as "smoking mirror," which is a metaphor for all that cannot be clearly seen in our ordinary states of perception.[8] Tezcatlipoca as the smoking mirror also refers to the obsidian mirror. In many ancient images, Tezcatlipoca is often wearing an obsidian mirror. Obsidian is a powerful, sacred stone revered in both ancient and modern Mexico. The many uses of obsidian in curanderismo include dreamwork, shadow work, healing, divination, protection, and psychic surgery. For some curanderx, obsidian is their primary instrument used for healing.

Mictlampa presides over the realm of our dreams. In the Anahuacan cosmovision, it is believed that each night when we dream, our energetic dream body (nahual) travels to the same place that we journey to when we die. Death is seen as an extended dream during which the spirit travels out of the body, and in Nahuatl the word *temectli* means "the dream," "the land of dreams," and "the one who died." When we are alive and dreaming, our spirit travels out of our body each night, but returns home to the body each morning. When we die, the spirit leaves the body permanently.

In death, the spirit travels through the nine levels of the underworlds, or inframundos. Each inframundo also corresponds to a level of our unconscious mind. The concept of the underworld is similar to what Carl Jung called "the shadow." The underworld relates to the parts of ourselves that are concealed from our conscious mind. Hidden in our underworlds are the parts of ourselves that we reject, don't like, or don't want to face. This includes our heavy emotions, negative repetitive patterns, painful ancestral stories, addictions, lack of discipline, and self-sabotaging behavior. However, the underworlds are also considered places of power because our hidden gifts and abilities also reside there. We can access and work with the material in our underworlds in many ways, including in ceremonies such as the limpia or in psychotherapy. In this tradition, working with the obsidian mirror is one of the primary ways to access the under-worlds. Another way to connect to our underworlds, which is accessible to all people, is to work with our dreams, as is covered in depth in chapter 13.

## CONNECTING WITH MICTLAMPA

To work with Mictlampa, face the north direction while praying, meditating, or doing healing work. Or conduct your rituals at midnight or outside under the moon. Since Mictlampa is the land of the dead, it is an energy to work with when you wish to connect to and honor your ancestors. A simple way to do this is to build an ancestral altar with photos of your beloved dead, flowers, candles, water, and other special objects.

Any kind of obsidian stone also brings in the energy of Mictlampa. One of the most powerful forms of obsidian is the obsidian mirror, although there are many forms of obsidian, including spheres, eggs, pencils, and knives. Obsidian is a strong stone that can bring up difficult emotions, so I recommend getting train-ing in how to work with it. The ideal time to tap into the energy of Mictlampa is midnight, so try doing your spiritual practice or ritual in the middle of the night.

Mictlampa is a powerful direction for healing, as its energy helps us see, understand, and cleanse our unconscious mind. Parts of ourselves that we don't like or accept are often stored in our unconscious. We can harness the energy of Mictlampa to help us face difficult situations and to see how we might be par-ticipating. Mictlampa also helps connect us to our dreams, and we can call this energy to our lives when we want to develop ourselves as dreamers.

## Huitzlampa (Rumbo Sur, South Direction)

**Huitzlampa** corresponds to the south direction and translates to "the place of Huitzilopochtli," the energy of the hummingbird warrior. Hummingbirds are small but mighty. They can fly thousands of miles without stopping. In the great migration of the Mexica tribes from Aztlan to Tenochtitlan (present-day Mexico City), a hummingbird guided them tirelessly for thousands of miles to their new home.

Huitzlampa relates to high noon and to the radiant energy of the sun, which powers all life on earth. This is the direction of children and youth, who naturally possess raw, vital energy. Huitzlampa gives us energy to fight for things we believe in, such as justice and equality. Huitzlampa provides to us the energy to protect the things we cherish, such as our families, our communities, and Tonantzin. The energy of Huitzlampa also conveys the warrior qualities of discipline and willpower. It gives us the strength to fight the battle within ourselves and to be warriors for our own healing.

In this tradition, Huitzlampa relates to the water element, the colors blue and green, and the number ten. Two important energies relating to water also reside in the south, Tlaloc and Chalchitlicue. Tlaloc is the energy of the rain, lightning, and thunder, and dwells in a mythical lush, green, fertile paradise called Tlalohcan. Tlaloc relates to agriculture because rain is essential to make plants grow. Tlaloc's companion is Chalchitlicue, "she of the jade skirt," who represents the essence of all terrestrial waters, such as lakes, rivers, and oceans. Tlaloc, as the essence of rain, can take the shape of four sacred waters: life-giving rain, hail, floods, and drought. Each of these four sacred waters corresponds to phenomena in nature, and they also correspond to emotional states within us. Healing water (gentle rain) is present when our emotions are balanced, and our lives can flourish. Hail relates to strong, destructive emotions that may not be fully expressed. Floods are powerful, overwhelming emotions that can cause damage to ourselves and to others. Drought is an absence of the natural flow of emotions, when our emotions are blocked and we don't allow ourselves to feel.[9]

## CONNECTING WITH HUITZLAMPA

To align with the energy of Huitzlampa, build your altar in the south or face the south direction when doing your healing work. Include on your altar a bowl of water or items that are blue and green. The energy of Huitzlampa is most active during the middle of the day, so you can harness its energy by doing your work in the afternoon.

# RITUAL: ACTIVATING OUR INNER WARRIOR

We all have experienced challenges in our lives during which we need to call on our inner warrior for strength. The challenge may be an external one, such as fighting discrimination we have faced in the workplace. Or the challenge may be internal, such as fighting our own addictive behaviors or negative repetitive patterns.

When you need to harness the qualities of Huitzilopochtli, such as strength, endurance, discipline, and willpower, a simple ceremony is to go outside around noon (or whatever time the sun is at its zenith in the sky). Face the south direction, give an offering to Huitzilopochtli, and say your prayers. Ask Huitzlampa for the qualities of a warrior that you need right now. Connect to the heat and power of the sun. Imagine yourself as a blue-green hummingbird with limitless power to face your challenges. The number associated with Huitzilopochtli is ten, so to optimize your prayer, repeat this exercise for ten days in a row.

## RITUAL: HEALING OUR INNER WATERS

The energy of Huitzlampa can support our emotional healing work. To heal ourselves, we need the strength, courage, and endurance of a warrior. Huitzlampa also corresponds to Tlaloc and Chalchitlicue and the realm of our own emotional waters.

One of my favorite ways to work with my inner waters is through the practice of herbal baths, or baños. In baños we connect directly with Chalchitlicue and her sacred waters. Chalchitlicue can help us connect to our emotions and bring them back into balance. Water helps us cleanse ourselves and release what is no longer serving us. I will share more in depth about herbal baños and give suggestions for practices to support yourself in chapter 11.

# The Cosmos

In Danza, after we greet the four sacred energies of Nauhcampa, we next gaze upward to greet the energies of the sky and of the cosmos. This includes the energy of the thirteen heavens, which house the moon, sun, planets, stars, and galaxies. Our ancestors carefully observed the effects these celestial bodies had on their lives. The original inhabitants of Mexico had highly sophisticated knowledge of astronomy, and many sacred sites such as the Pyramids of the Sun and the Moon at Teotihuacan were built to be in alignment with celestial events.

## CONNECTING TO THE COSMOS

Take time to watch the movement of the sun across the sky. Observe the moon through its cycles of new, waxing, full, and waning. Gaze at the constellations. Sleep outside under the stars. Make offerings and meditate on any of the celestial energies.

# Tonantzin

## CANCION HUEY TONANTZIN

Huey Tonantzin, Tonantzin
Huey Tonantzin.
Ipalnemohuani
Noyolotl Tatzin/Noyolo paqui
Tlazohcamati
Tonantzin*

After greeting Nauhcampa and the cosmos, in Danza ceremonies we end by kneeling on the ground and honoring our Mother Earth Tonantzin. This relationship is at the foundation of the healing work of curanderismo, and as you remember your ancestral medicine, keep finding your way back to the earth.

## CONNECTING WITH THE ENERGY OF TONANTZIN

Find a safe, quiet space outside. If you are indoors, create an altar with items to represent Tonantzin, such as plants, flowers, stones, fruit, or even dirt. You can sit, stand, or even lie down on the earth.

Start by grounding and feeling the energy of the earth. If you are outside, meditate on the natural world around you. Reflect on all the ways that Tonantzin supports and nourishes your life. Give thanks and make an offering to express your gratitude. Ask Tonantzin what you can do to honor her.

---

* Traditional Nahuatl prayer song.

# Corazón/Heart/Teyolía

Although not a common practice in Danza, in the Curanderx Toolkit class, after greeting Nauhcampa, the cosmos, and Tonantzin, we take a moment to be still, place our hands on our chest, and feel our heartbeat. We greet the divine spirit that dwells inside the corazón, the heart, the teyolía, of each person in the class.* We honor the spark of life that makes our heart beat and animates our bodies. We feel how the sacred energies of Nauhcampa, the cosmos, and Tonantzin all come together in each one of us. We recognize our place in the universe and in the continuity of life. We feel our ancestors standing proudly behind us and know we are the answer to their prayers. We sense the presence of the future generations, the children, the youth, the babies, and those yet to be born. We feel our sacred responsibility to ourselves, our ancestors, our families, our communities, the earth, and future generations.

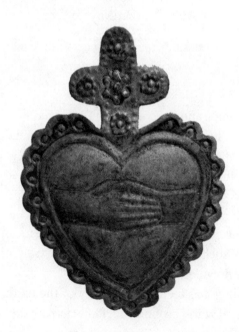

---

* The teyolía will be explained more in the section on the four energetic bodies in chapter 10.

## MEDITATION: HONORING YOUR DIVINE SPARK

Place your hands on the center of your chest. Breathe into your hands. Feel the beating of your heart. Acknowledge the divine spark that gives you life. Honor the unique spark that is you! Feel how the beating of your heart connects you with love to the heartbeat of Mother Earth, the cosmos, all of life. Honor your sacred responsibility and your sacred purpose. Give thanks for the miracle of your life!

# Embodied Experience

Building a relationship with Nauhcampa and the forces of the universe is an embodied practice. We cannot learn about these cosmic energies simply through books or lectures. Instead, we must regularly engage with the cosmic forces by using our bodies, hearts, minds, and spirits. Each person will develop their own relationship to the cosmic forces. I am sharing some of my experiences and observations, but each of you will develop your unique understanding. Practice. Experiment. Observe. Remember that our ancestors developed this philosophy through thousands of years of studying the natural world and also by observing human nature. Nothing can replace lessons learned from our embodied experience. Our embodied experience as healers is the foundation for all of the work we do. As we learn to connect to the energy of the cosmos, we can bring that energy to our healing work. Letting go of our ego and tapping into forces beyond ourselves are essential parts of nuestra medicina.

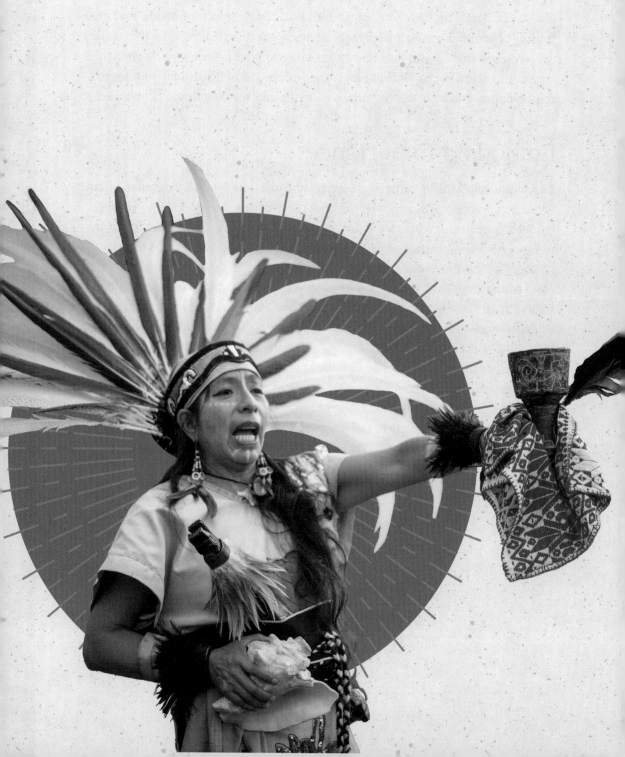

## SPOTLIGHT

# Patricia Chicueyi Coatl
## (she/her/ella)

> "Learning about the Nahuatl/Toltec/Anahuacan cosmovision is of the utmost importance on the path of curanderismo, lest you hurt yourself or others with ceremonial techniques used without proper understanding of the foundation of that knowledge. By studying this cosmovision, you will be honoring the millions of ancestors who nurtured the relationship with the sacred elements thousands of years before we were born."

Born and raised in Mexico-Tenochtitlan, Patricia Chicueyi Coatl comes from a long and strong lineage of Nahuatl temazcaleros, pulqueros, and growers and protectors of huauhtli (amaranth), tlaolli (corn), etl (beans), and metl (agaves). Her parents and grandparents were Nahuatl native speakers who raised her in a lovingly disciplined Nahua way. The first ancestral medicine taught to her was to relate to one another with the utmost respect. Her parents taught her at an early age to be responsible for all her acts, words, and decisions. She received her first limpia at age four from her dad when he cleansed her with tobacco smoke. Her mom taught her how to talk to and care for plants, and how to use them for food and medicine. From her abuelita she learned about the loving power of the Tlecuil (Nahua hearth), and her abuelito taught her to plant and harvest corn and beans.

Patricia Chicueyi Coatl is a danzante and leads Calpulli Huey Papalotl, a Danza Mexica circle that shares Anahuacan ceremonies, traditions, and culture in Huchiun Ohlone territory. As a scholar of Anahuacan traditions and practitioner of Mexica traditional knowledge, she has dedicated her life to sharing her ancestral knowledge (matiliztli) and supporting her community.

When I met Maestra Chicueyi Coatl, I was excited to meet a strong woman leader in the Danza community, and became a member of Calpulli Huey Papalotl.

I was privileged to attend her calmecac sessions* where she taught us calpulli members the history, cosmology, culture, and philosophy that informed Danza Mexica. She is also a regular guest teacher in the Curanderx Toolkit class. I have immense gratitude and respect for her huge and generous heart. She is a warrior who shares her ancestral wisdom with countless people and continuously offers herself to help heal her community.

## PATRICIA CHICUEYI COATL SPEAKS:

The Danza tradition taught me that carrying a sahumador puts us on the path of the healer. Each sahumadorx is a healer and has the responsibility to care for and protect our community with limpias, rezos, sobadas, cleaning the space, offering healing cantos for our community and for the sacred energies.

My advice for people on this path is to be extra respectful, by always asking permission. When working with plants, ask the plant permission to work with her. The plant might say no, and you have to understand that no is no. When interacting with macehualtin (human beings), always ask permission to come into their circles, regardless of how big or small those circles are. Do not take what is not yours, and even if they taught you some healing ceremonial technique, be cognizant that it doesn't mean that you can now use it for your own benefit. Part of being respectful is also knowing your curanderx lineage: who are your teachers, where do they come from, who are their teachers and where do they come from, etc. If you teach, the first thing you should do is openly share your lineage.

I am blessed to know that I am never alone because I have a profound connection with las Señoras y Señores de la Tierra; with the spirit of the plants; with the spirit of the trees; with Ehecatl, the spirit of the wind; and with the spirit of the fire. I know they listen to me and nurture me, I know I can always depend on them, and I know I can always honor them by offering my tears, cantos, palabras, and rezos.

---

* *Calmecac* is a Nahuatl word that means "house of the lineage"; these were places in Mexica society for training and higher education, primarily for sons of nobility.

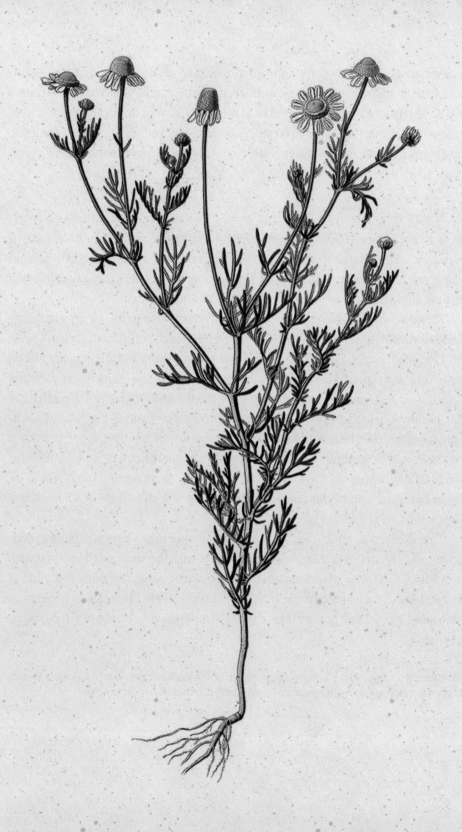

# CHAPTER 6

# Herbal Allies

## MY LOVE POEM TO PLANTS

Queridas plantas
Gracias
For always sharing
For always supporting
For unconditional love
For continuing to help us humans
Even when we've forgotten how to respect you.

Thank you for growing in my garden
For returning every spring
For persisting even in drought
For feeding the soil
For flowering
For offering yourselves
To bees
To butterflies
To birds.

Thank you for your healing aroma.
Sweet citrus of melissa
Pungent yarrow
Savory rosemary
Spicy thyme, oregano, basil.

Thank you for your beauty.
Golden cempohualxochitl
Pink trumpet tobacco flowers

Bold magenta bougainvillea
Bright orange and yellow nasturtium.

Thank you for your medicina.
You are the magic
In a cup of hot tea
Nourishing bodies
Calming nerves
Relieving pain
Releasing tension and stress
Relaxing to sleep
Fighting that cold
Cleansing unwanted energies
Healing all the cuts, scrapes, bites and wounds
Soothing my sadness,
Depression
Heartbreak.

Each time I walk in my garden
Greet your familiar faces
I smile
Touch your leaves
Inhale your scent
Breathe more deeply
Remembering
Vast epochs of time
Human evolution
Inextricably woven with our plant relatives.

You are our elders
Ancestors
Our interconnected relationship
Encoded in our DNA.

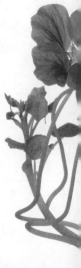

My gratitude is immense
Beyond words
Please accept my humble offering
To honor you
To listen to you
To protect you
To never take too much
To care for the places where you grow.

I sing praises to each one of you
Growing in my garden.

I call you by these names
Yarrow
Melissa
Sage
Mugwort
Yet what do you call yourselves?

                             Do you have a name for me?

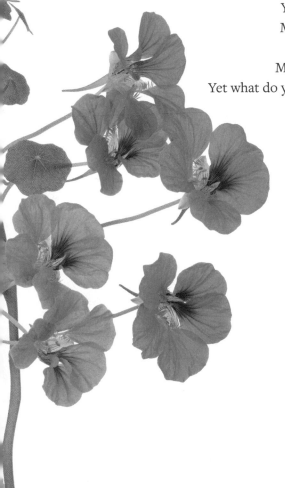

# La Casa de la Medicina

The moment you enter the home of a curanderx, you will immediately sense something special, magical, and healing. You will be embraced by a symphony of colors and aromas: vibrant bouquets of flowers, freshly harvested mint, rosemary, ruda, or sage mingling with the smell of pungent chili and a pot of frijoles simmering on the stove. Altars decorate the house, carefully constructed on tabletops, cabinets, and kitchen counters, and in front of the fireplace. Each altar has a unique purpose and is artfully designed with candles, crystals, photographs, copalero (popoxcomitl, incense burner), bundles of herbs, feathers, and instruments. In the kitchen you might find bundles of herbs hanging to dry. Amber and cobalt-blue bottles full of herbal tinctures line the shelves of the medicine cabinet. In the pantry, you may discover mason jars full of plants soaking in alcohol or vinegar.

# Learning to Love Plants

> Plants tell their stories not by what they say, but by what they do.[1]
>
> —Robin Wall Kimmerer

It is hard to describe the feelings of fondness, love, and gratitude I have for the plant beings in my life. I began this chapter with a poem to capture the depth of those emotions. As humans, we are used to feeling love and affection for other human beings. For many, this love can extend to our animal friends as well. Yet how can we learn to love a plant?

Plants differ more from us than do animals, so developing a relationship with them requires more subtlety. Plants do not have eyes or ears or hearts. They do not move around like humans, animals, insects, and birds. Plants are sessile, which means that they are permanently rooted in one place.

For humans who have been separated from their Indigenous consciousness, it may be easy to assume that since plants do not share common characteristics with the animal kindom,* they lack intelligence. However, quite the opposite is true. Plants are extremely intelligent. They not only share with us the same five senses of sight, sound, touch, taste, and smell, but they actually possess fifteen more senses![2]

We can learn to love plants simply by spending time with them. As healers, we build our connection to plants as we begin to consciously interact with them. As we take walks in nature, as we tend to our gardens, as we cook or make medicine with plants, over time our relationship to plants will blossom (pun intended!).

The more I learn about plants and the more I strengthen my relationships with them, the more I am convinced that they possess unconditional love for us humans. Despite all the harm human beings have inflicted on the earth, plants are still here to nurture and support us. Plants give us food, clothing, and shelter. The herbal medicines of the plant world help our bodies stay healthy and heal us when we've been sick or injured. Herbs can help us relax and sleep, and they can also give us energy when we're feeling depleted. They can bring calm when we are feeling stressed, and they can lift our spirits when we are depressed. Herbs are very effective in treating trauma, which in curanderismo we call susto. They can help call the soul back into the body. Herbs comfort us when we are suffering from heartbreak or loss. Herbs assist and support us human beings in all stages of life, from birth to death.

As human beings, we carry the memory of plants in our DNA. All of our ancestors have been interacting with plants for countless generations. Our ancestors used plants for food, shelter, and clothing; in ceremony; and for medicine. Before our ancestors could go to a drugstore to buy aspirin for a headache, they learned to identify which plants growing around them could be helpful in relieving pain. The genetic memory of our plantcestors lives in our bones and blood.

Take a moment to pause and think about the ways plants have supported your life. Is your home built from trees? Is your clothing made of cotton? What is on your dinner plate? What is in your medicine chest? What plants are growing in your garden or in your neighborhood? Do you have a favorite tree you like to visit? Is there a place in nature that brings you a sense of peace and calm?

As we open our minds and hearts to the plant world, we begin to recognize

---

* I prefer the word *kindom* to the standard *kingdom* because it doesn't impart a patriarchal and hierarchical bias.

all that they give us each day, unconditionally. As we take in the generous gifts from the plant kindom, it is natural to begin to feel care and to love them. You don't have to work hard at it!

# Plant Knowledge in My Family

There are many ways that people learn about herbs in the tradition of curanderismo. For many, their families use herbal remedies at home, such as té de manzanilla (chamomile tea) to help with sleep or a cup of yerba buena (spearmint) tea for a stomachache. Many of my students and colleagues have shared stories with me of how herbs were used in their family home. For others, due to colonization, immigration, and assimilation, these traditional remedies have not been a part of their households.

I did not grow up with any herbal traditions from the Mexican part of my family. My mother and her siblings grew up in Detroit, Michigan, in the 1940s and 1950s and, due to a variety of circumstances, assimilated into American culture. They did not learn to speak Spanish, and they were not strongly connected to their father's Mexican traditions.

My family maintained their connection to plants through gardening. My Mexican grandfather, Jesus Garcia Delgado, always kept a small garden in his backyard, where he grew tomatoes and chilis. When I first traveled to Guanajuato, Mexico, to meet my Mexican relatives, I found out that they were campesinos who grew corn and avocados. Both of my parents also loved to garden. My Polish American father planted redwood trees and built a koi pond in our backyard. My mother starts each day going out to her garden to greet her plants. She grows dozens of varieties of roses as well as other flowers, fruits, and herbs. Together my parents transformed their backyard into a lush, thriving wildlife habitat and sanctuary. I believe that this ancestral memory lived on in both of my parents in their instinctual connection to growing plants. Although I come from a family of gardeners, the practice of using plants as medicine was not passed down to me.

# Falling in Love with Herbal Medicine

I discovered herbal medicine unexpectedly as a young adult when my sister, Jenny, invited me to come with her to the Northern California Women's Herbal Symposium.

That weekend, I was taught to identify a few medicinal herbs that grew like weeds around the land. *Plantain, chickweed, cleavers*. I learned to make herbal oil infused with pungent, sweet lavender. I discovered I could transform this herbal oil into a salve by putting it on the stove on low heat and adding a little beeswax. I was introduced to passionflower and scullcap, two herbs to help me sleep. (I tended to suffer from insomnia.) In the herbal marketplace, I bought my first herbal tincture, a blend to heal acne by supporting the liver, made from the roots of burdock, yellow dock, and dandelion. In the evenings, women gathered around a campfire and sang and danced by moonlight.

By the end of the weekend, I was totally in love with the plants. I felt that I had come home to a world I did not even know existed. My heart knew that this was what I wanted to do with my life. I had tucked in my backpack a flyer from a woman teaching herbal classes back home in Huchiun/Oakland. I was ready to sign up and begin my lifelong journey with the plants.

# Herbal Medicine in Curanderismo

There are many ways to work with herbs in this tradition without having been formally trained as an herbalist. An herbalist/hierberx is someone who prescribes herbs for treatment of various physical, emotional, and spiritual conditions. My education as an herbalist includes decades of training from teachers of different backgrounds, including curanderas, acupuncturists, and Native American and Euro-American herbalists. I weave together all the knowledge I have learned, but at its heart my practice is rooted in curanderismo.

The practice of herbal medicine in curanderismo is in no way homogenous. There exist regional differences, variations between diverse cultural groups of Mexico and different approaches in each family or teaching lineage. Each hierberx, depending on their cultural background, will have different ways of viewing the human body in health and disease. They will have different names and uses for plants. Hierberx from Indigenous and other nonwesternized backgrounds will be trained in a medical theory that is particular to their culture or tribe. Their understanding of the human body and disease may differ from those who are trained in a more western medical model of herbalism. Yet the common factors for all hierberx is a thorough knowledge of the plants, a thorough knowledge of the human body, and an understanding of the factors that influence human health and also those that contribute to sickness and disease.

## Philosophy of Hot and Cold

In curanderismo, as in many traditional systems of herbal medicine, qualities of temperature are attributed to each plant. The temperature of plants is a component of what herbalists of many traditions call the plant's energetics.* The energetics of a plant relate to the way it affects the tissues and organs of the body. Plant energetics can also relate to the way the plant moves energy in the body or the way the plant affects our emotional state. Not only does each plant have its own energetics, but so does each individual person and each illness. The art of herbal medicine is in choosing the right plant or plants to balance the energetics of the person and of the illness or imbalance that is presenting in them.

The temperatures of plants fall on a spectrum. Some plants are slightly warming (cinnamon); some are hot (cayenne pepper). Some plants are cooling (dandelion root), and others are cold (aloe vera). Plants can also possess different or even opposite qualities of temperature depending on the part of the plant used or the form in which it used. For example, cold yerba buena tea is cooling and refreshing on a cold day. Yet a cup of hot yerba buena tea will heat up the body and induce sweating.

In traditional Mexican medicine, food, herbs, emotions, and illnesses are all assigned a degree of hot or cold.** Heat in the body feels hot and inflamed. Fevers, rashes, redness, and irritation are all caused by excessive heat. Cold in the body feels heavy and stuck, and inhibits movement. When there is cold in the body, the blood is not circulating properly, which leads to stagnation that can cause swell-

---

* Plant energetics also include the way the plant affects water/moisture in the body. A plant can be described as moistening, drying, or somewhere in between.

** Although, according to Mexican historian Alfredo López Austin, who wrote *Textos de medicana náhuatl*, there exists much variation between different Indigenous communities and even between individual people as to what is considered hot or cold.

ing, pain, and lack of mobility.[3] Anger is seen as hot; fear and sadness are cold. When treating a person with a condition or illness, we use plants that harmonize the degree of hot and cold in the body. For example, if someone is consumed with anger, giving them hot, spicy food may aggravate their condition. Instead, we may choose a plant that is calming and cooling, such as melissa. If someone has chronic back pain, they will benefit from a baño of romero, which will warm the body and dispel the coldness stuck in the back.

The roots of the philosophy of hot and cold in curanderismo pre-date the arrival of Europeans. Our ancestors observed the dualities in nature: the cosmic dance between day and night, sun and moon, earth and sky. The sun and stars are hot; the moon, the clouds, and the earth are cooling.[4] As ancestors observed these phenomena in nature, they noticed that these same forces were at play in the human body.[5] As systems of herbal medicine evolved worldwide over thousands of years, our herbalist ancestors developed highly sophisticated ways of treating illnesses based on their understanding of hot and cold in the universe and in the human body. Many of the treatments my maestras have shared involve removing excess cold or heat from the body.

## Comparison between Herbal Practices

For the past few decades, the popularity of herbal medicine has grown in the United States, and many herbal schools exist throughout the country. Historically in these schools, much of the material taught about herbs comes primarily from a Euro-American (primarily white American) perspective. I was motivated to search out the herbal practices of my Mexican ancestors because it was something never taught to me in herb school.

I have spent a lot of time thinking about the differences between Euro-American herbalism that is typically taught in American herb schools and the herbal traditions from Mexican curanderismo. One thing that was surprising to learn was

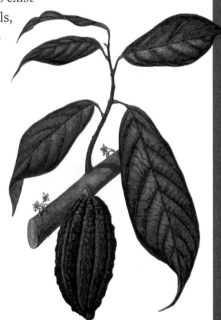

the similarities between both traditions.* Due to the history of colonization, both are influenced by European science, medicine, and culture, so these traditions sometimes share a similar language when talking about plants. For example, in Euro-American herbalism, the concept of "herbal actions" is used to describe how the healing properties of plants work on the body. Some common herbal actions are anti-inflammatory (an herb that decreases inflammation), diuretic (an herb that increases urine output), or diaphoretic (an herb that causes sweating). Although the concept of herbal actions is derived from Euro-American herbal medicine, I have heard these terms used by Mexican curanderas, and I will also use them in this book.

Similarities also exist in the plants that are used in both traditions. This includes many medicinal plants that came to the Americas from other parts of the world, including rosemary, rue, chamomile, and basil. Furthermore, many plants that are indigenous to Mexico, such as chocolate, chilis, epazote, and agave, are also used in both traditions. Before Spanish contact, there were over two thousand documented medicinal plants used in the Aztec empire, and many of these native plants continue to be used today.[6] Finally, many of the same genus of plants grow across different continents. One of my favorite examples of this are plants in the genus *Artemisia*. *Artemisia vulgaris*, or mugwort, is a cherished European herbal remedy. *Artemisia argyi* is a primary herb used in traditional Chinese medicine as moxa. The *Artemisia* native to California, *Artemisia douglasiana*, is used by Native Californians. Across Mexico and the Southwest, a primary herbal remedy is estafiate, or *Artemisia ludoviciana*. Across these different continents and cultures, the *Artemisia* plants are often used in similar ways.

However, differences also exist between the practice of Euro-American herbal medicine and herbal medicine in curanderismo. In Euro-American herbal medicine, especially as it is practiced in the twenty-first century, herbs are often viewed primarily from a perspective of biomedical science. The understanding of medicinal plants is reduced to only seeing them as a mere collection of chemical

---

* Euro-American herbalism is commonly called "western herbalism," a term I don't particularly like. To use this term implies that globally there are only two bodies of herbal knowledge: that which comes from the "west," meaning Europe and the United States, and that which derives from Asia. Entire continents with rich and ancient herbal traditions, such as Africa, are excluded. Moreover, this term ignores the legacy of colonization and the fact that much of American herbalism has been borrowed or stolen from Native American traditions. Yet for the purpose of this book, *western herbalism* refers to Euro-American herbal traditions as has been typically taught in most American herbal schools in the past few decades.

constituents that can interact with the biochemistry of the human body. The chemical constituents of plants are called phytochemicals, and the impact of these phytochemicals on the human body has been the subject of much scientific research.

If someone has a headache, a westernized herbalist may recommend taking a tincture of willow bark. Willow is high in salicylates, chemical compounds that reduce both pain and inflammation in the body. In this way, the phytochemicals in willow bark help relieve the person's headache, similarly to taking an aspirin. Aspirin contains a similar compound called acetylsalicylic acid, which is derived from willow.[7]

Likewise, from the perspective of Euro-American herbal medicine, herbs can also be used to address psychological ailments, such as depression, that are rooted in biochemical imbalances in the body. Often this relates to the levels of neurotransmitters such as serotonin or dopamine. To treat depression, an herbalist may recommend *Hypericum perforatum*, commonly known as St. John's wort.[*] This herb has the ability to inhibit the reuptake of both serotonin and dopamine, thereby increasing the levels in the body.[8] In this way, *Hypericum* works similarly to some selective serotonin reuptake inhibitors (SSRIs) and can be used to treat mild cases of depression.[**]

In curanderismo, we also use plants to address physical or emotional conditions, and many of us also study the phytochemistry of plants. At the same time, we understand that plants are not just a collection of phytochemicals but also sentient, intelligent beings. We consider the plants to be our teachers, spiritual guides, and helpers in our healing work. In curanderismo (as in many Indigenous traditions), we take time to study the more subtle spiritual and energetic healing properties of plants and then apply this knowledge to our work. When we are rooted in an understanding of the spiritual and energetic healing properties of plants, we can work with plants in many different ways to address the conditions

[*] *Hypericum* was a very sacred plant in ancient Europe, traditionally used for protection and magic. It normally puts out its first blooms right around the summer solstice. By naming this plant St. John's wort, the Catholic Church co-opted this sacred plant by naming it after the patron saint of the summer solstice, St. John the Baptist. I personally prefer not to use this colonized name for this plant.

[**] *Hypericum* can be a useful herb for depression, but it has many contraindications and interactions with medications. Please consult with an herbalist to determine whether this is a safe herb for you to take.

from which people suffer. In the case of treating depression, a curanderx also may prescribe hierba de San Juan (St. John's wort) as a tea. In addition to prescribing the tea, they may also give their client a limpia to help release negative energies absorbed from the environment. These energies may have been contributing to the depression, so removing them is an essential part of the treatment. Another curanderx may treat the same client by prescribing a baño of white flowers, since they know it will help release stagnant emotions/aires. The curanderx knows that these blocked emotions might lead to feelings of being depressed and that for the depression to be fully healed, they will help their client address and release these blocked energies.

# Herbal Allies

> Talking to plants is one way of talking directly to Spirit.
> —Rosemary Gladstar

Each curanderx develops a special relationship with particular plants. These plants may be a key ingredient in her spice cabinet, or a tea she drinks regularly, or they may be the herbs she is cultivating in her garden. Our favorite herbs, which I call our herbal allies, are like our best friends. Our herbal allies are our trusted guides in all the healing work we do.

We build relationships with our herbal allies by incorporating them into our daily lives. We can cook with our herbal allies or use them as medicine. We can sit quietly in a garden and practice listening to the quiet voices of plants. We can invite our allies into our sleeping space and dream with them. Our relationship with plants is at the heart of our work.

It is important that we create a reciprocal relationship with our herbal allies. The plants give us so much: oxygen, food, medicine, clothing, shelter, and beauty. How can we give something back to them? A good way to give back is to tend to plants in your garden. We can also make offerings of prayer, food, song, dance, or art to our herbal allies as a gesture of our gratitude.

# Discovering Your Herbal Ally

Finding your herbal ally is not a hard or complicated process. Often your herbal allies are already a part of your life in some way. Identifying your herbal ally is a way to bring more awareness to the relationship that already exists between you and your plant friends.

✺ Open your eyes. Notice what herbs are already around you. What are your favorite spices that you use for cooking? What herbs do you prefer for tea? What go-to herbal remedies do you keep in your medicine cabinet? What plants are growing around you? What herbs do you love to cultivate in your garden?

✺ Open your heart. What plants do you feel drawn to? Is there a certain plant that always catches your eye when you go out in nature? Is there a plant whose aroma you find intoxicating? What herbs make you feel good when you take them? What plants are you dreaming of? What plants did your ancestors use?

✺ Open your mind. Sometimes you do not choose your herbal ally, but your herbal ally chooses you. Learn to listen to your intuition and open yourself to the quiet whispers of the plants. Sit still. Be quiet.

✺ Talk to the plants. Offer a song or prayer to the plants in your garden. Ask for their guidance and support. Ask for your herbal ally to reveal itself to you.

How do you know you've discovered your herbal ally? Listen to your body. You will feel happy and uplifted being near your ally. You will feel excited working with your ally or even talking about your ally to a friend. Your ally will touch your heart with a deep knowing. Sometimes, meeting an herbal ally feels like falling in love.

Once you have identified your herbal ally, take some time to learn some basic information about it. The most important thing to know at first is whether it is safe to ingest. In the world of plants, there are many beautiful plants that are also toxic. If you are drawn to a plant that is poisonous, you may spend time with this plant, but please do not ingest it. Some plants, such as poison oak, are also not safe to touch.

Plants that we label as "toxic" or "poisonous" are not bad plants. All of them have something to offer the ecosystem, and many of them can be used as medicine by experienced practitioners. For example, poison oak grows in soil that has been disturbed in some way by human use, and it is a protector of the forest.

Many herbs are safe for most people but need to be avoided in certain circumstances, such as pregnancy or postpartum. Other herbs need to be avoided (or used only under the supervision of an experienced herbalist) by elders, children, or people on certain medications or with certain diagnoses. In herbalism, we call these herbal contraindications. Make sure you do your homework to identify whether your herbal ally is safe for you to take as an herbal medicine.

We all have many herbal allies. Just as we each have a circle of human friends, each of us also has a community of herbal allies. Our herbal allies work together to support us physically, emotionally, mentally, and spiritually.

## Building a Relationship with Your Herbal Ally

Getting to know your herbal ally can be fun! The first step in building a relationship with your herbal ally is to engage with it regularly. Once you know you have an herb that is safe to take internally, make all kinds of herbal medicine with your ally. Bathe with your ally. Cook with your ally. Cultivate your ally in your garden. Spend time with your ally in nature. Meditate and dream with your ally.

Give thanks to your herbal ally. Make offerings to your ally and let it know how much you love and appreciate it in your life. Write poetry about your ally. Make art inspired by your ally. Praise your ally with music, song, and dance.

In the beginning, however, I would advise that you do not do too much research about your plant. Instead take time to be with the plant. This helps you experience the plant in a genuine way without any preconceived ideas about it. Sometimes our logical minds can get in the way of our listening to our intuition. There is a plethora of information about the medicinal use of plants in books and on the internet, but your ally may show you something about itself that cannot be found in books.

# Herbal Ally Story: Tobacco

Tobacco began speaking to me years ago and has become one of my most important teachers. Over the years, I have received direct instructions from the plant on how to be in relationship with it.

One hot summer day, I was at a liquor store buying tobacco to bring to a ceremony for offerings. In the store, I looked around at the boxes and bags of loose tobacco and cartons of cigarettes. Nearby were shelves of beer, wine, and hard alcohol. Around me, people, mostly people of color, were filling their shopping carts with cartons of cigarettes and cases of beer.

In a flash, I heard this voice in my head saying, "THIS IS NOT YOUR PRAYER!" It felt like a sudden splash of cold water to my face. I was startled and flooded with waves of sadness and anger. In a moment of spiritual clarity, I received this download from tobacco:

*How could I be praying for the health of my communities while supporting businesses that make profit selling poisons to Brown, Black, and Indigenous folks?*

*How could I pray with tobacco that had been grown not with a prayer but with greed for profit?*

*How could I pray with tobacco that was grown not with love and respect for Mother Earth Tonantzin but with harsh chemicals that pollute the earth and water and become poison in the human body?*

My head felt hot, and my temples were throbbing. I abandoned my cart and rushed out of the store without buying anything. In that moment, I made a commitment to honor this message and to change my behavior.

I decided to start growing my own tobacco.

As I embarked on my assignment to grow tobacco, I was intrigued because although it is considered to be a very sacred plant, its true nature was hidden beneath the layers of colonization and exploitation. As an herbalist, I know that each plant has a different personality and a different purpose. I was curious to learn more about the personality and spiritual essence of tobacco.

Tobacco is a sacred plant to many of the Indigenous people of the Americas. It has many uses for ceremony, prayer, doctoring, birthing, and healing. Tobacco is a messenger or conduit to the spiritual world. As an offering, tobacco opens the channels of communication between humans and the spiritual world, and its smoke carries prayers to the four winds of the universe.

When Europeans settled and colonized Turtle Island and its Indigenous inhabitants, they also managed to co-opt and exploit this sacred plant. As lust for tobacco grew in Europe and Asia, tobacco cultivation became a major force of colonization. The cultivation of tobacco also played a key role in the enslavement of African people. Many plantations where Africans were enslaved were tobacco plantations, and enslaved people were forced to work long, grueling hours in tobacco fields. The free labor of slavery fueled the exponential growth of the tobacco industry.

In modern times, the multimillion-dollar tobacco industry continues to harm people and the earth. Commercially cultivated tobacco contains over seven hundred toxic chemicals, including arsenic, lead, formaldehyde, and benzene. Cigarette smoking is one of the highest risk factors for disease, including cancer, heart disease, COPD, and other respiratory diseases. In the United States, one in five deaths is related to smoking tobacco. A study conducted by several health organizations from around the world found that tobacco production has many detrimental impacts on human health and leads to environmental problems such as pollution, deforestation, loss of biological diversity, and soil degradation.

*How could I uncover the true spirit of tobacco buried under years of human abuse and exploitation of this sacred plant?*

The more I reflected on my desire to grow tobacco, the more I realized that I had received an assignment from the spirit of tobacco. This plant, sacred to many people, including my own Diné and Mexican Indigenous ancestors, was demanding my attention, urging that I take the time to know it as a sacred being, not just as an object that has been mistreated and misused for centuries.

I started by researching all that I could about growing tobacco. The scientific name for the tobacco genus is *Nicotiana*. I found a seed company that sold different types of *Nicotiana*, and I ordered some to plant in my garden. I discovered that the genus comprises many different species, which vary in size, shape of the leaf, color of the flower, and the climate in which it prefers to grow.

The first year of my tobacco-growing project, I planted two varieties of tobacco in my garden: the classic *Nicotiana tabacum*, which is most widely used in commercial cultivation, with long, narrow leaves and creamy pink trumpet flowers; and the smaller *Nicotiana rustica*, with short, dark-green leaves and mustard-colored flowers. *Nicotiana rustica* is native to the Southwest and is also called Hopi tobacco or Aztec tobacco.

Some friends also shared tobacco plants with me: *Nicotiana sylvestris*, with fragrant, white tubular flowers, and a *Nicotiana* of unknown species native to Oaxaca, Mexico, which grows as tall as a tree, with bright pink flowers well loved by pollinators. I discovered that in the mild Mediterranean climate of California's Huchiun/East Bay, tobacco is quite easy to grow. It loves sun and rich soil. It doesn't like frost, yet that rarely occurs in Oakland. Tobacco plants have thousands of tiny black seeds, which spread widely. I've often found dozens of baby tobaccos that have self-seeded close to the mother plant.

I was inspired to plant many tobacco plants so that I had plenty to give away to friends. I felt as though tobacco was also instructing me to help educate others about its true nature and bring awareness about the right use of this plant. When my baby tobaccos were large enough to transplant, I happily gave them away to my students and to other interested people at ceremonies, gatherings, and birthdays.

I am on a lifelong journey with my herbal ally tobacco. I cannot imagine my life or my work without the presence of my herbal allies. They continue to teach me, guide me, and support my path as a healer. I hope that by sharing my story, I have inspired you to build relationships with your own herbal allies.

I end with a prayer/poem to my beloved ally tobacco.

Tobacco
Tobaco
Piciyetl

Abuelx plant
Planta sagrada
Master healer
Spiritual messenger

Ancestors knew
Right relationship with you

To pray
To purify
To heal
To birth
To communicate with Creator

Your smoke carries our prayers
To the four corners of the universe

Help us to remember your sacredness
May we help you to grow
May the bees enjoy your flowers
May we hang your leaves to dry
May we share the harvest
May we save your seeds and give them away
So all can propagate

May you be free
From the historical prison of abuse
Removed from your sacred place
Co-opted by greed
Tainted by the legacy
Of crimes against humanity
Colonization
Slavery
Genocide
Pollution
Toxicity
Illness
Death

That is not your true nature

May we learn to be
In right relationship
With you

May ancestral memories
We carry in our bones and blood
Be liberated

So that we may
Once again
Treat you
As our beloved elder
Queridx abuelx
With love and respect
Con amor y respecto

Tlazohcamati

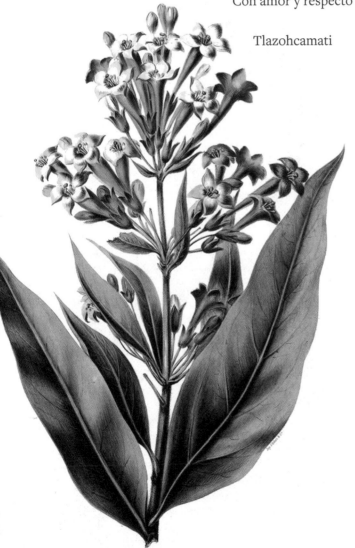

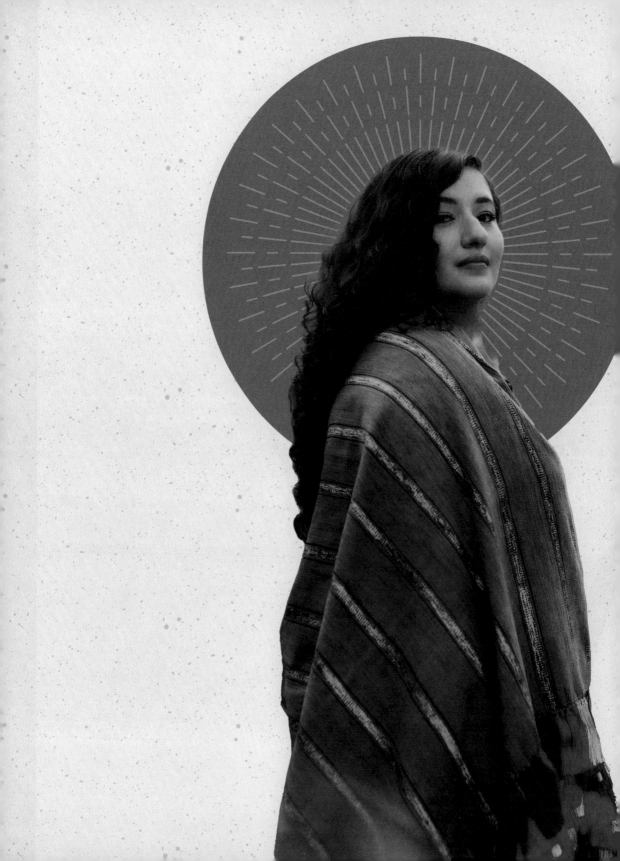

# Berenice Dimas
## (she/her/ella)

> "The path is open to you. It is a path waiting for you. It is a generous path to those who are called and those who accept the calling. This path will guide you, challenge you, test you, expose you to depth you have never experienced or known. It will show you how to listen deeply, how to be present, how to trust. This path will teach you accountability and consent. This path has the potential to remember, heal, and will set pieces of yourself free."

Born in Tenochtitlan (Mexico City) and raised on Los Angeles/Tongva lands, Bere is a full-spectrum birthworker (doula), an herbalist, and a midwife in training. She was raised by a mother who always kept an herbal garden and used remedios caceros (home remedies), such as limpias with huevos, massage, and herbal baths. People in the community sought out her mother for healing support, mostly postpartum care. When Bere got older, she began to help her mother with some of these practices to treat her two younger sisters. I met her when she became my student, and I soon recognized her gifts as a healer and teacher. When I needed to take a break from teaching to tend to my health issues, Bere accepted the responsibility of teaching the Curanderx Toolkit class. Bere is also the visionary founder of Hood Herbalism, which offers herbal education and training to the BIPOC community.

## BERENICE DIMAS SPEAKS:

My mother taught me how to build relationships with plants through her own practice of tending to and connecting with them. She also taught me how to support them when they got sad, how to communicate with them, how to water them properly, and how to make home remedies for ailments they also experienced.

I would not identify what I do as "curanderismo," and that is a teaching that was passed down from my mom. People have identified what we do in my family and my work in the community as curanderismo, but this work is more than anything a way of life. They are practices that have existed in my family for many generations.

One of the biggest blessings of this medicine has been finding the capacity and strength to recover pieces of myself. To recover pieces of my family's past. Healing generational trauma. Accessing generational and ancestral wisdom. Growing. Transforming. This journey is an ever-evolving process of learning. I am blessed with a path that allows me to share the beauty of plants and their medicine with people in the community. I am eternally grateful to these ways for the way they guide and open paths for me. I love how they connect me with people, places, lands, and energies. This medicine has been so gentle and loving in helping me also learn how to trust in what I know and what I feel.

Plants are always present when I support birthing families. During the prenatal time, it is important for me to have flowers at every session. There are pregnancies that are very smooth for people, and there are pregnancies that bring up a lot for people. I place flowers close to where we check in or do our sessions. The flowers are my supporters and help hold the space. I've been taught by my mom, maestras, and abuelas that flowers uplift vibrations. They offer tranquility and absorb stagnant energy. Although I use many other plants in my practice during the prenatal period, flower medicine is present consistently.

When a person is in labor, I like to offer the birthing person a special homemade chocolate. I ethically source, hand-roast, grind, and prepare the chocolate. Chocolate is one of my ancestral medicines, and it has been used in birth for generations. During labor, chocolate helps release endorphins, which work together with dopamine, serotonin, and oxytocin. The chemical collaboration that chocolate induces supports the birthing person's heart, brain, and emotional well-being. The endorphins help reduce the perception of pain that people experience during labor by promoting relaxation.

My mother was someone in the community who supported families specifically during the postpartum period. One thing she taught me was that regardless of the birth outcome (which includes abortion, miscarriage, and stillbirth), the most important support we could offer physically to the birthing person was to help bring warmth back into the body. During labor the pores open, the bones move, muscles stretch, ligaments expand. In emergency situations, cesareans and other surgeries are needed, which all cause cold to come into the body. My mom always told me that "el parto es una experiencia fría y se tiene recuperar el calor." She shared that birth is a cold or cooling experience for the body, so it is important to help bring back that warmth. My favorite herbal practices to support someone during the postpartum period are baths, teas, steams, warming foods, and massage. There are special formulations for each type of care, but all of them involve warming plants.

I apply ancestral healing knowledge in all areas of my life. This knowledge is the energy that guides my path. It is the energy I am accountable to. It is the energy I go to for support and guidance. It is the energy that I am deeply committed to uplifting, protecting, and passing down to our future generations.

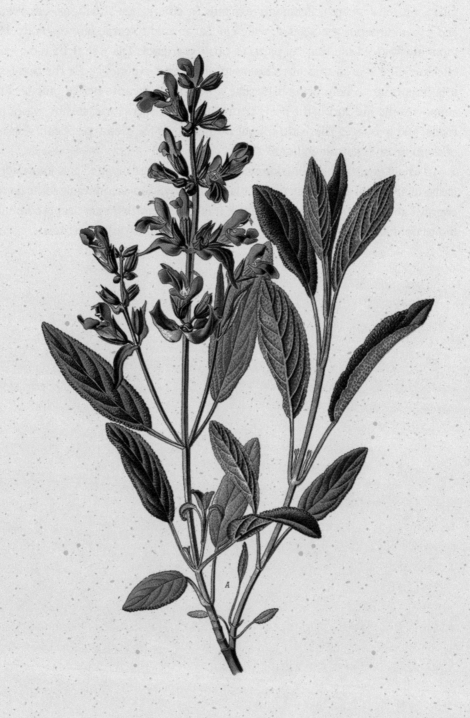

# CHAPTER 7

# Tending to Our Gardens

If you visit the garden of almost any curanderx in Huchiun/the Bay Area, you will find plants that are well loved by curanderx everywhere: a proud ruda plant guarding the entrance to the house, a hedge of pungent romero, and sunny golden flowers of pericón. Perhaps you'll encounter a stand of cheerful manzanilla, vibrant orange cempohualxochitl flowers, or the aroma of sweet-smelling yerba buena. The space is alive with birds, bees, butterflies, and ladybugs. Simply being in the garden is healing.

## The Importance of Growing Our Own Medicine

In a capitalist society, we are conditioned to believe that we need to pay for everything that we require for daily life. Many of us have lost the self-sufficiency of our ancestors, and we shop for our food, our clothing, and our medicine. However, traditionally curanderx grew or gathered most of their own medicinal herbs. Their herbal apothecary was sourced from what they could grow in their gardens or what they could harvest from the wild.

For many curanderx, the foundation of our healing work begins in our gardens. We need freshly harvested herbs to use for our limpias, baños, and medicine making. To obtain these herbs, we need to either grow them ourselves, gather from a community garden, or harvest them from natural spaces (although I mostly advise against wildcrafting).

If you don't have access to a yard to grow your plants, one solution is to learn how to grow herbs in pots and containers. Also, many herbs can be grown well indoors. Another excellent option is to connect with your local community garden. Community gardens exist in different cities and neighborhoods across the state. All the community gardens that I know of welcome volunteers in exchange for the opportunity to grow and harvest plants for your food and medicine.

Our gardens not only supply medicine but also are places of healing. My garden held me while I wept over the death of my father. My garden calmed me when I was suffering susto from receiving a cancer diagnosis. When I'm feeling ungrounded or spaced out, I sit or lie in my garden until Tonantzin and the beauty and aroma of the plants bring me back into my body.

By tending to our gardens, we awaken our ancestral memory. As we get our hands in the dirt, as we sow and nurture seeds into leaf, flower, and fruit, we activate this ancient knowing from inside us. When we grow our own herbs, we learn to build a reciprocal relationship with the plants. The relationship between a curanderx and their plants is at the heart of their work. We learn to take care of the plants that take care of us. We learn how to nurture our herbal allies with good soil, compost, and the right amount of sunlight and water. We talk to our plants as they grow. We sing to our plants when we harvest their leaves, flowers, berries, or roots for medicine. We tell our plants how we will be using their medicine and ask them to offer their healing power to the medicine that we make. In turn, the plants we grow know us and work with us. The medicine that we make from plants we have grown is more powerful and effective than anything we could buy in a store because it is infused with our love, care, and respect.

As we grow our own herbs, we also strengthen our connection to Tonantzin. We learn about the cycles of the seasons and the stages of the moon. We observe the ecosystem of our garden and discover the creatures who live there: bees, butterflies, moths, worms, ladybugs, and more. We learn which plants attract beneficial pollinators. Our garden is our classroom, and it teaches us daily.

My garden has taught me to honor the power of Tonantzin. Each day, the universe shares freely all the elements we need for life: water, air, soil, and sunlight. Tonantzin transforms these elements into roots, leaves, branches, flowers, fruit, and seeds. She creates beauty. She builds habitats. She nurtures and feeds the insects, animals, and birds.

 In my garden, I have witnessed the miracle of seeds, each tiny one containing all the intelligence and genetic information it needs to grow. I have planted and watered seeds and waited for days or weeks until a tiny green sprout pushes up from the soil, reaching for the sunlight. I have watched my seedlings grow into stands of chamomile or calendula. Sometimes, as in the case of my tobacco plants, my seedlings outgrow me and reach heights over six feet tall.

My garden has taught me patience. Sometimes my seeds don't sprout. Other times my seedlings are eaten by snails. Some plants, such as echinacea, require years of growth before they can be used as medicine. During times of drought, my heart aches as I watch my plants struggling to adjust to the hot, dry conditions.

Learning to grow our own herbs is also critical to the survival of many medicinal plants. For the past few decades in the United States, the popularity of herbal medicine has skyrocketed. As the demand for herbs increases, herbs are being exploited for profit, which has had a devastating impact on medicinal plants and the ecosystems in which they grow. Around the globe, people are facing shortages of medicinal plants due to overharvesting and destruction of their natural habitats. We are facing an unprecedented threat of shortage or extinction of some of our most valuable medicinal plants.[1]

To ensure the availability of all our beloved plants for future generations, I encourage everyone to learn to grow their own herbs. In many parts of California, we are blessed with a mild climate and a year-round growing season. Start growing your medicine on a small scale. Buy one herbal seedling from your local garden supply store and tend to it. As you advance, try growing one plant from seed to harvest, and share your plants' seeds with others so that they can grow these plants too. For support, connect with local growers in community gardens.

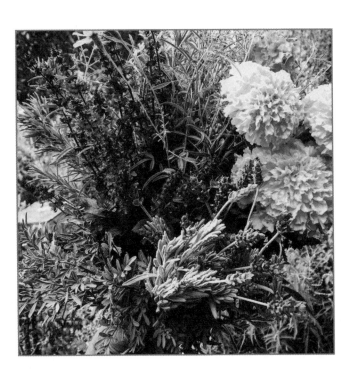

# Curanderx Herbs for California Gardens

California has many microclimates. The plants I am sharing here grow well in most coastal and inland environments, although growing conditions in mountain and desert ecosystems may be different. For each plant, I will share a brief description of the growing conditions.

## Sage/Salvia/Huitzihzilxochitl

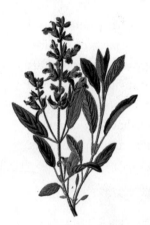

*Salvia* spp

The genus of plants called *Salvia* includes over a thousand species, which can be found growing on many continents around the world. One of the most well-known species in this genus is culinary sage, *Salvia officinalis*, which is native to Europe but grows well in gardens throughout the Americas. Sage species plants grew in Mexico before the arrival of the Spanish invaders, and the medicinal use of sage was documented in the Códice de la Cruz-Badiano. One Nahuatl name for the *Salvias* is Huitzihzilxochitl, which translates to "hummingbird flower."[2]

### MIRTO/COYOXIHUITL TLAZTALEUALTIC

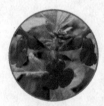 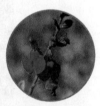

*Salvia microphylla* (mountain sage)
*Salvia greggii* (baby sage, autumn sage)*
**Energetics:** warming

Hummingbirds love mirto, and planting it will attract hummingbirds to your garden. Hummingbirds love mirto's long, tubular red flowers, shaped perfectly for a hummingbird's beak. Mirto is a common shrub that likes sun and well-drained

---

\* *Salvia microphylla* and *Salvia greggii* are both commonly called mirto. They are similar in appearance and medicinal use and are often used interchangeably. Both are native to Mexico. The monograph on coyoxihuitl tlaztaleualtic that appears in the Códice de la Cruz-Badiano has been interpreted to be about *Salvia microphylla*.

soil. It is both drought and frost tolerant and can be propagated from seeds or cuttings. In Nahuatl this plant is called coyoxihuitl tlaztaleualtic, which translates to "pink coyote grass."[3]

## MEDICINAL USE

According to the Códice de la Cruz-Badiano, mirto was used medicinally to treat fatigue and was also used as a sleeping aid, especially for children. To support sleep, bathe the child with mirto before bed and also place branches of it under their pillow.

Mirto is used traditionally to treat susto, espanto, and mal de ojo. As a tea, it helps calm crying children. Similarly to ruda, mirto is also used to treat earaches by placing a leaf in the ear.[4]

People in Puebla use mirto for menstrual cramps, to treat vaginal bleeding, to increase fertility, and as a postpartum bath. The Totonacs, Zapotecs, and Mixtecos all work with mirto to treat digestive complaints such as gas, bloating, diarrhea, colic, stomach infections, and empacho. A topical application of mirto is used to treat skin conditions such as rashes and pimples.[5]

## CORDONCILLO/MEXICAN SAGE/TOCHOMIXOCHITL

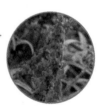

*Salvia leucantha*
**Energetics:** cooling and heating

Mexican sage is a very common shrub in gardens throughout Huchiun/the Bay Area. Its long stalks of fuzzy purple flowers add a splash of bright color to gardens. The flowers are surprisingly soft and pleasing to touch. It grows easily in Huchiun/Bay Area gardens and requires very little care. It is drought tolerant, but cannot handle a hard frost. It loves a hearty pruning and can be propagated from cuttings.

Although it grows ubiquitously in Huchiun/the Bay Area, Mexican sage has been underutilized by herbalists and curanderx. It had grown in my garden for years, yet I did not know about its medicinal use, nor did I know of any herbalist using it as a medicine. I would mainly use it for decoration and cut the colorful purple flowers to add to bouquets.

In 2012, I hosted Mexican curanderas Doñas Doris Ortega and Felipa Sanchez at my house. One morning, Doña Doris, who is an expert hierbera, led me on an herb walk in my own garden. She pointed out the different plants she knew (which was most of them!) and described to me their use. One of them was the Mexican sage plant, which she said was good for "female hormones" (for people who menstruate). Doña Enriqueta also uses it for birthing people to strengthen and tone the uterus. She also recommends it as a vaginal wash.[6]

In Morelos, cordoncillo is also a plant to cure sicknesses of aire and often mixed with cinnamon and fennel and prepared as a hot tea. This combination is also used to treat coughs and pain in the chest and lungs. Cordoncillo mixed with basil, sage, and epazote and a little pinch of salt is a treatment for stomachaches. Historically it has also been used to treat alopecia (hair loss) and dizziness.[7]

### SUGGESTIONS FOR USE OF MIRTO AND CORDONCILLO

Take internally as a tea, tincture, or flower essence. Use externally in limpias, baths, steams, salves, and liniments.

### CONTRAINDICATIONS

Avoid in pregnancy. Do not use while nursing, because sage can dry up breast milk.

## Yerba Buena/Mint

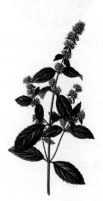

*Mentha piperita* (peppermint)
*Mentha spicata* (spearmint)
**Energetics:** cooling (when prepared cold) and warming (when drunk hot)

The common name yerba buena refers to many different herbs, most of which are in the mint or *Mentha* genus.* I will focus on two of the most commonly used mints, peppermint and spearmint.

---

* Yerba buena is also the common name of a native Californian plant, *Clinopodium douglasii,* which is not in the *Mentha* genus, although it does have similar medicinal properties to mints.

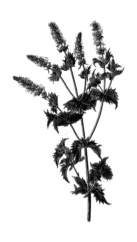

In Mexico and across the world, mint is one of the most well-known and widely used herbal medicines. At least one mint plant (*Mentha canadensis*) is native to Mexico. Many mint species are native to Africa, Asia, and Europe and were brought to Mexico by the colonizers. Yerba buena and spearmint grow well in full sun to part shade. Both plants prefer rich soil and regular watering. Some gardeners prefer to grow mint in containers because it can spread profusely and crowd out other plants. I prefer to let my mint grow wildly in the garden, and experiment with all the different ways I can use it as food and as medicine. Mint can be propagated by cuttings of either the root or the stem or by dividing the roots.

## MEDICINAL USE

Fresh mint is invigorating and refreshing. Its sweet and pungent scent is both familiar and comforting. I often use fresh mint for my limpias. Its energy is lightening and brightening and can help relieve heavy energies such as sadness and depression. Mint is stimulating and energizing to the mind and helps bring our awareness to the present moment.

Mint is high in volatile oils, which are the essential oils that give mint its pleasant aroma. These volatile oils are anti-inflammatory, pain relieving, and decongestant. The essential oils are most concentrated in the fresh plant. The oils of the fresh plant can be easily absorbed into the skin with direct contact. A fresh sprig of mint rubbed on the temples can help with a headache. A sprig of fresh mint may be rubbed on the belly to relieve pain or discomfort in the digestive system. Another great way to receive the benefits of mint's essential oils is with an herbal steam. As a steam, fresh mint can help relieve headaches, hay fever, and sinus infections.

A cup of yerba buena tea is a common remedy to soothe a tummy ache. All species of mint are beneficial to the digestive system. As a tea or tincture, mint helps ease cramps and spasms in the digestive tract and can be useful to relieve gas, bloating, and nausea.

Mint has different medicinal properties depending on if it is drunk hot or cold. A hot infusion of mint tea is a remedy for colds, flu, and fever. Hot mint tea is diaphoretic, which means it will heat up the body and increase perspiration. A cold mint tea can be both delicious and cooling. Fresh mint also is a great addition to cooking. It can be made into a pesto and can be added to fruit or vegetable salads, soups, or beverages.

## SUGGESTIONS FOR USE

Take internally as a tea or tincture, or eat as food. Use topically in limpias, baths, steams, sprays, and liniments.

## CONTRAINDICATIONS

Use with caution in pregnancy. One species of mint, called pennyroyal, causes uterine contractions and can cause miscarriage.

# Estafiate/Mugwort/Iztauhyatl

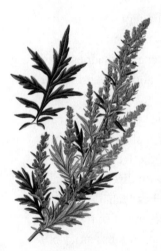

*Artemisia vulgaris* (shown)
*Artemisia douglasiana*
*Artemisia ludoviciana*
**Energetics:** cooling

There are many species of estafiate. *Artemisia vulgaris* is native to Europe but widely cultivated in North America. *Artemisia douglasiana* is native to California and the western US, and *Artemisia ludoviciana* is native to North America. Estafiate is a hearty plant that is easy to grow in many different conditions. It is drought tolerant, grows well in all kinds of soil, and can grow in sun, shade, or part shade. Estafiate grown in full sun makes stronger medicine.[8]

Once you establish it in your garden, estafiate will propagate itself by extending its horizontal roots, called runners. To grow from seed, sow seeds in the early spring, or propagate from cuttings or by dividing the roots.

## MEDICINAL USE

Indigenous groups of Mexico, including the Mexica, had been using estafiate for hundreds of years before European contact, and it is one of the plants documented in the Códice de la Cruz-Badiano. One translation of the Nahuatl name, Iztauhyatl, is "water of the sacred energy of salt." Estafiate is a sacred plant of Tlaloc, the divine energy of water, and is also associated with lightning. It is used in ceremony, healing, and divination.[9] In some regions, only elders are allowed to give limpias with this plant.[10] Estafiate continues to be one of the most important and commonly used medicinal plants throughout Mexico and the Southwest.[11]

Estafiate tastes very bitter, and its bitter flavor is a key to its medicinal properties. Bitter herbs benefit the digestive system by activating digestive juices and increasing peristalsis. As a bitter plant, estafiate supports many digestive issues including stomachaches, intestinal cramps, gastritis, and diarrhea. It is often combined with ruda, manzanilla, or yerba buena to treat digestion. A traditional remedy for parasites is to mix it with epazote.[12] Estafiate is also antimicrobial, which means it protects the body against bacteria, viruses, and fungi. It aids with colds, flu, and gastrointestinal infections. It can be used topically to treat fungal infections of the skin.

Estafiate is one of the most important remedies for empacho. Empacho is thought to be caused by a blockage of food in the intestines and is a common folk diagnosis in curanderismo.[13] Symptoms of empacho include stomachache, nausea, lack of appetite, constipation, or diarrhea. According to Doña Enriqueta, empacho can be caused by eating too much, eating spoiled food, or eating food that was poorly prepared.[14] Empacho can also be caused by eating too quickly, combining the wrong kinds of food while eating, or eating while upset or angry.

Estafiate is an emmenagogue, which means it stimulates the uterus. It can promote menstruation and ease cramping. Because estafiate stimulates the uterus, it should be avoided in pregnancy so as not to induce miscarriage.

Estafiate is also used in limpias to treat such conditions as mal aire, susto, and mal de ojo. In an herbal spray, mugwort can be used to purify a space. It is one of the ingredients I often include in my limpia liniment. It is also a powerful dream herb (see chapter 13).

## SUGGESTIONS FOR USE

Take internally as a tea, tincture, or vinegar. Can be used topically for limpias, baths, steams, sprays, or salve.

## CONTRAINDICATIONS

Estafiate should be avoided in pregnancy and nursing. It is a strong herb, so start with a low dose (five to ten drops of tincture or one cup of tea). Use with caution when working with children and elders. May be contraindicated for certain health conditions or with certain medications.

# Romero/Rosemary

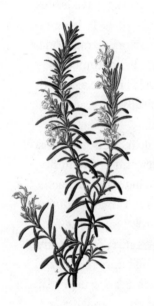

*Salvia rosmarinus*\*
**Energetics:** warming

Native to Asia and the Mediterranean region, romero loves full sun, tolerates drought, but cannot handle extended freezing temperatures. It tolerates poor soil and is resistant to many pests. When you first plant rosemary, it needs regular watering, but once it is established, it needs very little water.[15] It can also be propagated by cuttings.

For first-time herb growers, I recommend romero because it is easy to grow. Many new herb growers feel anxious that they will make a mistake and their plants will die. It is hard to kill this plant. It will grow well in pots and in the ground. It enjoys regular pruning, so once you have an established plant, you will have plenty of it to harvest for your medicine.

---

\* Until recently, rosemary's botanical name was *Rosemary officionalis*, but the plant was reclassified as a member of the sage genus in 2017.

## MEDICINAL USE

Romero is carminative, which means it supports digestive functioning and can help ease gas and bloating. It increases blood flow to the brain and can be used to improve both concentration and memory. The oil rubbed on the temples can help relieve headaches.

Romero is warming and stimulates the body's blood flow. A cup of hot tea can increase circulation and warm up cold hands and feet; an herbal steam can help alleviate sinus congestion and headaches. Inhaling the scent can be helpful with depression and sluggish energy.

Romero is great for both skin and hair. As a hair wash, rosemary can help increase circulation to the scalp and be beneficial for dandruff and hair loss. Used topically on the skin, rosemary can help disinfect and heal wounds and skin infections. Doña Enriqueta uses rosemary to help expel a stuck placenta.[16] Fresh rosemary can be added to many vegetable and meat dishes.

Romero is commonly used in limpias. It has strong warming energy, which activates and releases stuck emotions. It is particularly useful to help relieve cold aires/emotions, such as sadness and fear. The pungent, comforting scent of rosemary also helps call the soul back into the body. When giving a limpia, I often give my client a sprig of romero and ask them to hold it near their nose and inhale deeply. I encourage them to imagine the medicine of romero circulating throughout their body, completing an internal cleansing of their aires. Its scent is invigorating and helps the lost parts of ourselves feel safe coming back home to the body.

Romero is used in baños to help release aires, warm the body, and relieve achy joints and muscles. High in essential oils, rosemary is great for topical applications such as liniments or salves. The volatile oils in rosemary are easily absorbed through the skin.

## SUGGESTIONS FOR USE

Take internally as a tea, tincture, or vinegar. It can be used as a spice in cooking. Use topically for limpias, baths, steams, salve, oil, or liniment.

## CONTRAINDICATIONS

Do not use in pregnancy.

# Marigold

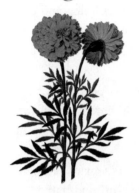

*Tagetes* spp

Plants in the *Tagetes* genus, called marigolds in English, are native to the Americas but have traveled around the world and have naturalized on many other continents. The *Tagetes* genus includes some of the most important plants used for medicine and ceremony in both historical and contemporary times.

## FLOR DE MUERTO/AZTEC OR AFRICAN MARIGOLD/ CEMPOHUALXOCHITL/

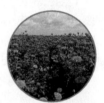

*Tagetes erecta*
Energetics: warming

Cempohualxochitl* symbolizes Mexican traditions unlike almost any other flower. With vibrant, puffy yellow or orange blossoms, it is an iconic part of Dia de los Muertos altars and celebrations. Its pungent, sweet scent immediately transports me to a place of reverence. It is native to Mexico and has been used in ceremonies and for medicine since long before colonization.[17] Cempohualxochitl is easy to grow from seed. It loves sun and well-drained soil, but can tolerate both clay or dry soils. It is drought and heat resistant, but cannot handle frost.[18]

## MEDICINAL USE

Cempohualxochitl has many healing qualities and is often used to treat digestive issues, such as pain, gas, empacho, colic, diarrhea, vomiting, and cold in the stomach. It supports the liver and works against parasites. It relaxes nerves and can help with insomnia. It benefits the hair and skin and can be used topically for rashes, sores, warts, pimples, and eczema. It benefits the respiratory system and is used for cough, colds, flu, bronchitis, and coldness in the lungs.[19] Doña

---

\* Multiple spellings exist for the Nahuatl name for *Tagetes erecta*, including cempasúchil, cempazuchitl, and cempaulxochitl.

Enriqueta uses it for menstrual cramps, for postpartum baths, and to help with lactation.[20]

Cempohualxochitl is an outstanding remedy for healing emotions. It brings brightness and hope when we are facing sadness, grief, and other heavy emotions. Its colors and aromas comfort us in the face of death and loss. In Puebla and Oaxaca, it is used in limpias to treat los aires, such as susto and espanto.[21]

## PERICÓN/YERBA ANIS/YERBA DE OFRENDA/ MEXICAN TARRAGON/YAUHTLI

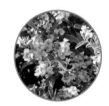

*Tagetes lucida*
Energetics: warming

*Tagetes lucida* grows as a perennial or annual, depending on the climate. It propagates easily from seed, loves full sun and well-drained soil, and can tolerate moderately cold temperatures.

The Nahuatl name of this sacred plant, yauhtli, translates to "an offered-up thing or incense" or "cloud medicine."[22] Pericón normally appears after the first rain and signifies the time of the season to start planting crops.[23] It corresponds to Tlaloc, the revered energy of the rain who also protects the fields from mal aire. Pericón was traditionally used as an offering to Tlaloc and also Chalchiuhtlicue (energy of terrestrial waters, such as oceans, rivers, and lakes) in central Mexico for centuries before European contact and use continues to the present day. Pericón is burned as an incense to communicate with ancestors and sacred energies. In Morelos, people construct crosses of pericón to protect their homes and crops on September 28. This date corresponds to the feast day of San Miguel, yet originally this time was to honor Tlaloc.[24] Crosses of pericón are also left at crossroads to enact "the sweeping of the roads," which prepares the fields for harvest and cleansing.[25] Offerings of pericón are also made to water spirits who dwell in caves nearby fields.[26] Nahua people decorated temples with pericón, added it to containers to store dried beans, and mixed it with chocolate to make a ceremonial drink.[27] Pericón has been used traditionally as an herb of protection from lighting and from drowning.

I first learned about pericón in a class with respected Mayan elder and curandera Grandmother Flordemayo, who calls it "the Grandmother Plant." She shared that pericón is a powerful being who guides other plants on how to use their medicine. Grandmother Flordemayo's teachings started me on a journey with the *Tagetes* genus (see the Grandmother Plant section, next).

## MEDICINAL USE

Since pre-contact times, *Tagetes lucida* has been used to treat "cold diseases," such as dampness, swelling, and phlegm in the body. Doña Enriqueta recommends pericón to treat conditions of aire and coldness, especially when the cold is located in the waist, chest, ears, or head.[28] She also uses pericón to treat menstrual cramping and scanty blood flow, and in baños to support fertility.[29] Other parteras use it to prepare birthing people for labor, to bless the expecting parents, and to bathe the newborn baby. Grandmother Flordemayo makes an oil of pericón to enhance meditation and spiritual work.

Pericón is a true pharmacy chest and also can benefit anxiety, depression, asthma, nausea, colds, flu, infections, pain, and many other conditions.[30] Pericón has a tarragon-like flavor and can also be used as a spice for cooking.

## MEXICAN MARIGOLD/MOUNTAIN MARIGOLD/ THE GRANDMOTHER PLANT

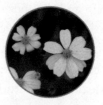

*Tagetes lemmonii*
**Energetics:** warming

*Tagetes lemmonii* is native to southern Arizona and northern Mexico and grows abundantly throughout the temperate regions of California. It is drought tolerant and resistant to many diseases, although it cannot handle frost. It can be started from seeds or from cuttings.

When I first received teachings about pericón from Grandmother Flordemayo, I realized that its sibling species, *Tagetes lemmonii*, grew in my front yard. It is a large bush with yellow composite flowers and a strong perfumy scent. In herbalism, often different species of the same genus of plants are used interchangeably. As an experiment, I decided to harvest some to bring to class and share with my students so that we could learn about its medicine collectively. I invited them all to take the plant home to work with in dreams and meditation.

When my students shared their encounters while dreaming with this plant, many of them reported powerful healing experiences.

As we continued to work with the plant, we saw a pattern emerge—it commonly brought dreams of mothers, grandmothers, and elder women, so frequently that we began to call it "the Grandmother Plant." For example, one of my students had a neighbor who was grieving the recent death of her grandmother. She felt sad because she hadn't connected to her grandmother's spirit in her dreams. My student offered her some of this plant, and that night she dreamed of her grandmother. I continue to work with this plant to help people connect to female ancestors in dreams.

## MEDICINAL USE

*Tagetes lemmonii* has actions similar to pericón, and is used to treat digestive issues. It grows abundantly in Huchiun/the Bay Area, where curanderx often use it for limpias. It can be used in baños for healing los aires and will turn your bathwater yellow. It is a powerful herb to use in meditation and dreamwork.

## SUGGESTIONS FOR USE OF ALL *TAGETES* SPECIES

Take internally as a tea, tincture, or vinegar, or add as a spice to food. Use topically for limpias, baños, steams, salve, oil, or liniment.

## CONTRAINDICATIONS

Do not take in pregnancy.

---

\* This name was also inspired by Grandmother Flordemayo, who also named its sibling species, *Tagetes lucida*, the Grandmother Plant. In this book, the Grandmother Plant is referring to *Tagetes lemmonii*. This is an example of how different plants can share a common name.

# Ruda/Rue

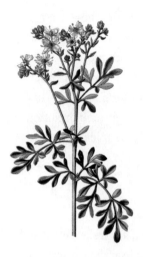

*Ruta graveolens*
Energetics: warming and cooling

Ruda is native to both North Africa and the Balkan Peninsula. It grows easily in many climates and thrives in full sun. It prefers well-drained soil, but can tolerate other kinds. Ruda is drought tolerant, but cannot handle extended freezing temperatures. It can be propagated by seeds, cuttings, or root division.[31] The ruda plant I have growing in my garden today is the great-great-great-great-grandchild of my first ruda plant. Every time I have moved, I have taken a cutting and planted it in my new home.

## MEDICINAL USE

Ruda is used for stomach pain, inflammation, and digestive issues caused by excess anger. To support digestion, it combines well with chamomile. It is used topically for both earaches and headaches. Ruda in combination with mint and epazote works for menstrual cramps, especially when caused by bathing in cold water or by eating overly acidic foods.[32] Ruda is also useful for regulating the menstrual cycle; it can also be used to accelerate labor and induce abortion.[33] Parteras use ruda mixed with chocolate to help the womb relax and to release the placenta after birth.[34]

Ruda has been used traditionally for parasites and headaches, and topically as a remedy for pain, inflammation, and insect bites. As noted, ruda is also an excellent remedy for earaches. To help relieve pain and inflammation in the ears, gently place a small folded-up leaf of the plant in your ear. Be careful not to insert it into your ear canal. To treat a child, soak a cotton ball in a ruda tea and place the cotton ball in the ear.

Mexican curandera Doña Doris Ortiz teaches that ruda is the plant of forgiveness. It helps us forgive ourselves and others. She teaches that ruda helps eliminate fear, clears our minds of persistent thoughts, and brings a sense of peace. She recommends either bathing with ruda or hanging a branch of ruda in the shower so that the water flows over the rue and onto your skin while showering.[35]

Ruda helps release both aires and negative energies, and is often used for cleansing and protection. I like to wear a sprig behind my ear for psychic protection or to use it in a liniment. Ruda is a strong plant that does not heal gently but delivers an herbal kick in the ass. Sometimes we need this kind of healing, but it can be uncomfortable. When used in limpias, ruda has the capacity to activate movement and release all of the aires. I find ruda to be too strong for many people, so I only use it in small amounts. I often prescribe a flower essence of ruda for people to use after they receive a limpia, so that they may continue the process of releasing their aires. I find the flower essence to be a gentle way to interact with this plant.

Ruda must be used with caution. Take internally in small doses, as large amounts can be toxic. Most of the teachings I have received about ruda recommend using only a tiny piece of the plant when taking internally. Ruda should not be taken internally during pregnancy, as it can induce miscarriage. Ruda contains volatile oils that when combined with sunlight can cause a rash much like poison oak. I highly recommend that when using the fresh plant topically, only do so over clothing and never in sunlight. Once I gave a limpia with ruda to a friend of mine in her backyard. The next day she woke up with a painful red rash all over her belly where I had rubbed her with ruda. I learned the hard way to be respectful and careful with this powerful plant!

## SAFE USES OF RUE

- Be careful about exposing bare skin to the ruda plant in sunlight. If you harvest ruda on a sunny day, wear gloves.
- Ruda can be toxic when taken internally, so only use in small amounts or under the guidance of a trained herbalist.
- Do not use ruda when pregnant. Some sources say to avoid in breastfeeding, but ruda also has been used traditionally to stimulate lactation.

# Pirul/Peruvian or California Pepper Tree

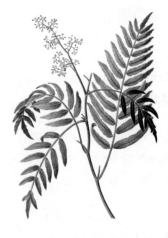

*Schinus molle*
Energetics: warming

Pirul is native to Peru, but is now grown widely in compatible climates throughout Mexico and California. Pirul is hearty and easy to grow and is actually considered an invasive plant in some parts of the United States. It is drought tolerant and grows well in various soil conditions, but cannot tolerate freezing temperatures. It can be grown easily from seeds; its seedlings are best planted in sunny areas. Pirul will grow into a tree twenty-five to forty feet tall, so plan accordingly when planting in your garden.[36]

A famous Mexican curandero named El Niño Fidencio (1898–1938) regularly performed healings under a large pirul tree. Thousands of people made pilgrimages to see him and to be healed under the tree, called El Pirulito, which also was considered to have great healing powers.[37]

## MEDICINAL USE

Pirul is a warming and spicy herb that increases circulation in the body. It is used topically or in baths to decrease pain in muscles or joints. It supports the digestive system and helps with gas, cramping, and bloating. It is used as a poultice or liniment to disinfect wounds, to stop bleeding, and for toothaches. Hot pirul tea is used to treat respiratory ailments such as cough and bronchitis. Parteras use pirul mixed with romero, ruda, and lettuce leaves for postpartum baths, and also apply a poultice of pirul on the breasts to stimulate lactation.[38]

Pirul is a very protective herb that is commonly used in limpias, the temescal, and other forms of spiritual cleansing. Doña Enriqueta uses it to treat los malos aires such as susto (shock) and mal de ojo.[39] Doña Doris Ortiz also recommends using pirul as a bath to remove negative energies and mal de ojo and to relieve tiredness and fatigue.[40]

Pirul branches and leaves are made into bouquets by themselves or combined with other plants. The pirul is dipped in water or sprayed with alcohol to help activate the plant's medicine.

## SUGGESTIONS FOR USE

Take internally as a tea, tincture, or flower essence. Use topically in limpias, baños, steams, salves, or liniment.

## CONTRAINDICATIONS

Avoid in pregnancy.

# Saúco/Blue Elderberry/Mexican Elderberry/ Xometl

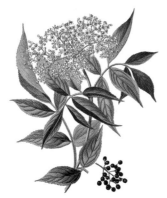

*Sambucus nigra* ssp. *canadensis*
(formerly *Sambucus mexicana*)
Energetics: leaves are cooling; berries are slightly warming.

Blue elderberry is a native plant that grows throughout California and across Mexico. It is a relative of the more widely known black elderberry, *Sambucus nigra*, which is native to Europe and the eastern United States. The genus *Sambucus* comprises twenty species that grow in temperate climates across many continents.

In nature, elderberry grows in many different locations from near the coast to high elevations. Elderberry will grow best in full sun or partial shade. *Sambucus nigra* needs rich, well-drained soil and plenty of water, but blue elderberry can tolerate many kinds of soil and levels of moisture. To propagate, start it from seeds or from cuttings.[41]

## MEDICINAL USE

Since antiquity, many people across the world have relied on elderberry as a trusted herbal remedy. The elder tree is a complete pharmacy in itself. The berries, flowers, and leaves all have medicinal properties. However, the leaves can be toxic and should only be used externally.

In Mexico, elderberry has traditionally been used to treat coughs, colds, respiratory infections, digestive problems, skin issues, parasites, inflammation, and many other afflictions. It is also a strong spiritual plant that has been used to treat susto, espanto, sadness, mal de ojo, mal aire, and soul loss. For these treatments, the flowers and leaves are used ceremonially in baths or in the temescal. Sometimes the flowers and leaves are massaged into the body with prayer, such as in Chiapas, where it is used in elaborate healing ceremonies.[42]

Elderberries are strongly antiviral. Elderberry is the top herb I use to both prevent and treat colds and flu. I personally start dosing myself with elderberry when I notice the first signs that I might be getting a cold; it can often back off the cold from becoming full blown. If I do get sick, I will continue to take elderberry throughout the course of the cold. I also recommend taking elderberry even if you feel well but are exposed to someone who is sick. Elderberry is a tonic herb and can be taken regularly during cold and flu season as preventive medicine.

In the past decade, medical research has shown that elderberry is an extremely powerful agent to protect the human body against flu viruses. Elderberries contain compounds called anthocyanidins, which are the phytochemicals that give elderberries their purple color. The anthocyanidins help strengthen the walls of our body's cells. With stronger cell walls, our cells are better protected against viral invasions.

## SUGGESTIONS FOR USE

Berries or flowers of blue or black elderberry can be taken internally as a tea, tincture, cordial, syrup, or honey.

## CONTRAINDICATIONS

Do not eat the seeds of blue or black elderberries, as they can be toxic. The berries of the red elderberry (*Sambucus racemosa*) are poisonous, so never ingest. Leaves of all *Sambucus* species are toxic if taken internally.

# Manzanilla/Chamomile

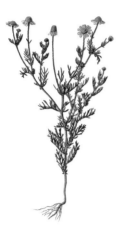

*Matricaria* spp
**Energetics:** warming and cooling

Manzanilla is a sunny, cheerful plant that is well loved by honeybees, ladybugs, and other pollinators. Manzanilla is easy to grow and prefers soil with good drainage and full sun. It helps protect other plants from pests and is a great companion plant for many vegetables and flowers. Manzanilla is also known as a "plant doctor," which means that it can help heal other plants. Plant a patch near any plant in your garden that needs support.

Manzanilla is easy to start from seeds, which you can sow directly in the soil or start in flats and transplant when they are bigger. It is an annual plant, which means its growing cycle is only one year. However, I have noticed that when I let my manzanilla plants go to seed, they reseed in my garden and pop up the following year.

## MEDICINAL USE

Manzanilla is a true panacea whose use as a medicinal plant dates back to ancient Egypt, Greece, and Rome. It has an affinity for the digestive system and can relieve gas, bloating, and cramping. It aids in relieving gastritis, ulcers, colitis, nervous stomach, colic, and irritable bowel syndrome. Manzanilla is soothing to the skin and is used to treat skin rashes; it is the first choice for treating dry, itchy, inflamed eyes. Manzanilla is tonic to the nervous system, is calming, and helps relieve stress, anxiety, and fear. It helps relax tension in the body and is also a wonderful aid for sleep and dreams.

## SUGGESTIONS FOR USE

Use flowers internally as a tea, tincture, or flower essence. Can be used in limpias, baños, steams, salve, or liniment. A cool manzanilla tea can be applied as a compress to relieve burning, red, or itchy eyes.

## CONTRAINDICATIONS

Manzanilla is generally considered safe for adults, pregnant people, children, elders, and pets. It may potentiate the effects of sedative drugs. It may be contra-indicated for people who are allergic to plants in the Asteraceae family.

# Melissa/Lemon Balm

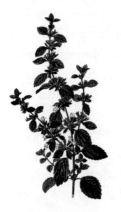

*Melissa officinalis*
**Energetics:** cooling

Melissa has been a steadfast ally of mine during all the years I have lived in Huchiun/Oakland. It grows robustly in Huchiun/the Bay Area and adapts to many different grow-ing conditions and climates. It is drought resistant, can thrive in full sun to full shade, and can grow in many types of soil. It can be propagated by seeds, cuttings, or trans-plants. Once it is established in a garden, it will spread.

Some people consider melissa to be an invasive weed. I look at it differ-ently. When a plant is growing in abundance in my garden, I take it as a sign that many people need its medicine. This has certainly been the case with melissa, as its healing properties are needed by many people in Huchiun/the Bay Area. The melissa in my backyard Huchiun/Oakland garden has provided countless people with medicine.

Melissa is in the mint family and looks similar to other mints such as yerba buena and spearmint. One of its signature characteristics is that it has a fresh lemony scent. Melissa's scent alone is healing! Simply grow it in your garden or in a pot on your porch so that your melissa plant will always be available for you to touch and smell. Inhaling the scent of a fresh sprig of melissa is relaxing and grounding. Its scent is also good medicine for sadness, grief, and depression.

## MEDICINAL USE

As an herbal nervine, melissa helps relieve stress, depression, and anxiety. It also decreases the nervous agitation that can accompany dementia. Like other plants in the mint family, melissa also supports digestion. It can relieve gas, bloating, and other digestive discomforts. A cup of melissa tea after a meal can help support digestive functioning.

Melissa is a traditional remedy to treat colds and flu. It has antiviral properties and can help relieve congestion and reduce the fever and pain that accompany a bad flu. The extract has been found in studies to be effective against different viruses, including rotavirus (stomach flu) and herpes simplex.[43] Taking melissa as a tea, tincture, or oil can help fight a herpes outbreak.

Melissa is one of the first plants I turn to for emotional support. Its sweet medicine gently tends to our emotions and works well with sadness, heartbreak, grief, anxiety, and depression. Once when I was working with melissa, I was sleeping with a fresh sprig of it each night. One night I awoke from a powerful and healing dream. In the dream I was connecting with an old friend whom I had been estranged from for many years. In the dream, we were able to connect in a loving way. I woke up with tears in my eyes and fullness in my heart. Melissa helped me access the old stuck grief around this relationship. With its support, I was able to open my heart and more fully grieve.

My first herbal teacher, Choctaw herbalist Karyn Sanders, taught that melissa has a particular affinity for healing sexual trauma. I have given it to people who have survived sexual abuse, rape, misogyny, and transphobia. Melissa also brings healing to people who have had abortions, miscarriages, hysterectomies, and traumatic birthing experiences. To work with healing sexual abuse, I prefer to use it as a baño. Soaking in its sweet medicine can bring a sense of comfort and peace. For healing trauma, it can be combined with other herbs such as cempohualxochitl, rose, or pericón. To repair boundaries that have been violated by trauma, combine with yarrow.

## SUGGESTIONS FOR USE

Use the leaves and stems internally as a tea or tincture. Use for limpias, baños, steams, salve, or liniment.

## CONTRAINDICATIONS

Melissa can inhibit thyroid activity, so it is contraindicated in hypothyroidism. Use with caution in pregnancy.

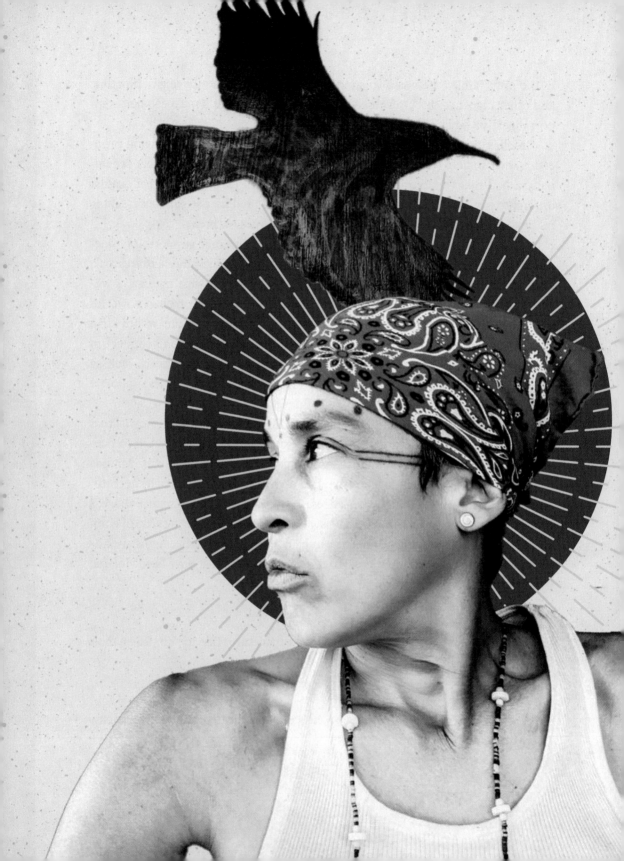

# SPOTLIGHT

# RaheNi Gonzalez
## (they/them/theirs)

> "As a displaced Indigenous person of mixed blood, the road to reclaiming my identity and these ancestral ways hasn't been easy. Distance from blood relatives due to colonial thinking on two-spirit people added a whole other layer to the challenges."

RaheNi Gonzalez is a two-spirit Boricua Taino ceremonialist, sacred artist, healer, and activist. They were born to Boricuan parents in occupied Lenape territory (Brooklyn, New York) and currently reside in Huchiun, occupied Ohlone territory (Oakland, California). RaheNi was raised by their Abuela Maria, who healed their nightmares, colds, and headaches with her bottle of Superior 70 Alcoholado (Bay Rum). RaheNi also remembers visiting the magical house of their great-grandmother and great-aunt who were Taino and practiced the old ways.

I met RaheNi decades ago when we were in our twenties in our shared two-spirit community, and we were raised together in this community of strong queer, two-spirit people. RaheNi brings impeccable artistry and deep spiritual groundedness to their work; they teach people how to create altars and ancestral remembrance and facilitate circles for queer, two-spirit, trans, and non-gender-conforming folks.

## RAHENI GONZALEZ SPEAKS:

In 1996, I was invited to a two-spirit ceremony where I began doing the work of healing colonial trauma and dismantling, within myself, colonized ways of thinking and being. I became very devoted to the Sacred Red Road and have had various teachers, elders, and mentors along the way. Through my involvement with Indigenous ceremonies, I gained much knowledge and developed a passion for creating altars/portals for healing and connecting with ancestors. I also have a passion for plants and enjoy making plant medicine, including salves for pain and various sprays for protection and cleansing.

When I'm having a hard time, the first thing I do is go to my altar, burn some medicine, light a candle, and communicate with my ancestors and guides and ask them for guidance. When I feel energetically off, I will give myself a limpia with the same Superior 70 Alcoholado my abuela used. The smell of it instantly calms and grounds me.

The plant used to make it is called malagueta. Its fragrance is similar to bay laurel, which grows in the hills of Huchiun. At the beginning of a walk there, I always ask permission to grab a bay laurel leaf so that I can inhale its scent as I walk among the trees. This simple act is deep medicine for me. Taking me back to those nights of being doused with alcoholado. Bringing me "home." So malagueta was the first plant I ever deeply connected to. I didn't know then that I would develop such a deep relationship to the earth and the plants.

Now, as an adult, my garden is my sanctuary, and it heals me on all levels . . . energetically, physically, and spiritually. From healing teas to gathering fresh herbs for limpias like lavender, pericón, romero, and ruda, my garden is the one-stop shop for healing! You can find a plant for just about any ailment, and this is very important for survival.

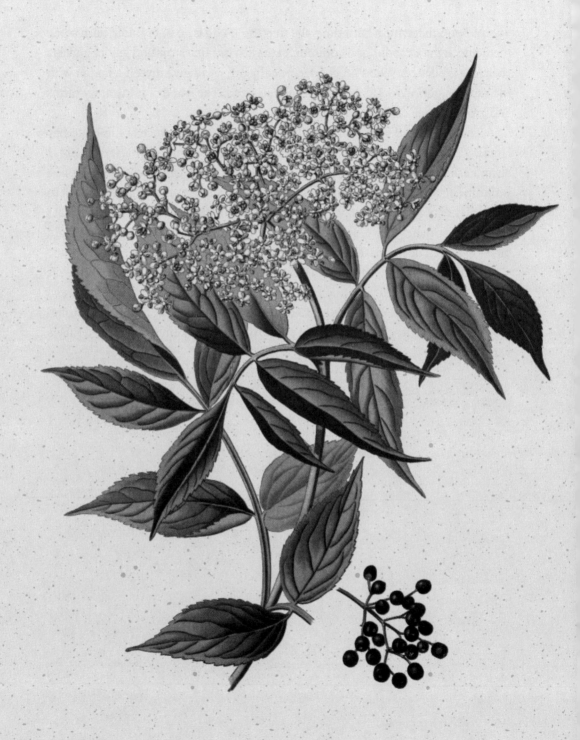

# CHAPTER 8

# Cultivating a Medicine-Making Practice

For many of us raised in modernized and westernized cultures, we are used to going to the store to buy our medicine. We are accustomed to thinking that our medicine comes from the pharmacy or the herb store. Many of us might not think of all the steps it took to make the echinacea tincture that is sitting on our kitchen counter.

Learning how to make our own medicine is enjoyable and empowering. Although the process may seem intimidating at first, many herbal medicines are quite easy to prepare. With a little bit of knowledge and some good recipes, you can fill your home medicine cabinet with your homemade tinctures, salves, vinegars, honeys, and cordials.

There are many benefits to making our own medicine. First, to make our own medicine requires us to work intimately with the plants. We learn about the plants in an embodied way, as we touch, smell, and taste the plants we are working with. The knowledge we gain about plants through this direct, hands-on, sensory experience with them is beyond anything that can be learned in a book. A book cannot convey the cheerful citrusy smell of fresh-cut melissa, or the way your fingers get covered in pungent sticky resin when processing yerba santa, or the effort and muscle power it takes to wash and finely chop up a fresh ashwagandha root.

We can save a lot of money by making our own medicine. What it costs to buy a two-ounce bottle of echinacea tincture could cover the cost of materials (the herbs, the alcohol, and the bottles) to make at least eight ounces of your own. When you grow your own herbs or gather herbs from your local community garden, you can leap over the gates that capitalism has closed to health and well-being.

Homemade herbal medicine also possesses a special, even magical quality. Homemade medicine, just like home-cooked food, contains the love, care, prayer, and intentions of the person who made it. I love taking medicine made by my herbal colleagues and students. I can taste and feel the care and magic that is in the bottle. This adds an element to the medicine that feels more powerful and healing than anything I could buy in a store.

# Creating Sacred Space for Medicine Making

One of the most important aspects of making medicine is our energetic space. The state of mind, heart, and spirit we are in becomes a part of the medicine, whether we are making a tea, a tincture, or a salve, or preparing herbs for a baño. I have learned never to make medicine when I am angry or upset. I do not want the anger to seep into my medicine.

At the same time, however, I do not expect myself to always be perfectly happy when making medicine. I have found that the process of making medicine itself can be healing and is an important part of the way we build relationships with plants. Working with the plants to process them into tincture has helped lift my spirits when I am grieving or when I feel depressed. To me, the process of making medicine is very meditative and calming. It helps me feel more grounded, peaceful, and connected to my body.

Some people prefer to make medicine alone and in silence. Others prefer to listen to music. I love making medicine in community because it is a great way to learn about the plants together. If I am making medicine with my students, we are mindful of our speech when we work together. We don't swear or gossip, and we avoid charged topics, such as politics. We share stories about the plant and what we are observing as we work with it. The spirit of the plant is a palpable force in the room, which influences our mood and conversations. Sometimes the plant makes us laugh and feel silly, and sometimes the plant can be sobering. Other times the plant elicits profound insight and revelations.

For me, medicine making is a ritual. I usually create a simple medicine-making altar where I light a candle and smudge myself with cedar, sage, or copal. I say a prayer to Tonantzin and thank her for providing me with these plants.

I also thank the plants and ask them to help me make a strong medicine for the people. I pray to my spirit guides and ancestors to help with the process.

Another factor that influences our medicine making is the astrology of the day and time we are making our medicine. Our medicine has a birthday just as we do! Our medicine will have the energetic imprint of the day it was born. I love making medicine on new moons, full moons, and on the solstices and equinoxes. I pay attention to which astrological sign the moon is in, as each sign has distinct qualities and gifts. I will also consult the Mexica calendar to know the cosmic energy of that day. All of these unseen cosmic energies become part of the medicine we make.

I encourage you to create your own medicine-making rituals. They will be shaped by your own personality, your own creativity, and your own particular spiritual beliefs and practices. There is no right way or wrong way to do it. The main thing I advise is to be mindful of making medicine when you are in a negative state of emotion, and to be mindful of your speech and thoughts. The creativity and ritual you put into your medicine making will become part of your medicina and be felt by everyone with whom you share it.

# Asking Permission

Sometimes when we ask permission of plants to harvest them, they will say no. Sometimes it is hard for us to listen and accept this message from plants. The "no" often comes as an inner knowing, or something may just feel off. We can also observe the signs in nature. One time when harvesting a plant with a group of people, I felt that we shouldn't be doing it. But I ignored my intuition because everyone else seemed to be OK. When we approached the plant, one of us slipped and fell. When we got close to the plant, a huge rattlesnake was coiled beneath it. Obviously, we took this as a sign that we shouldn't be picking the plant. When we all talked afterward, it turned out that many of us also heard the "no" from the plant, but ignored it.

# Making Herbal Tea

Drinking tea is one of the oldest and simplest ways to ingest medicinal herbs. All you need to make tea are herbs and water. Most people are familiar with drinking tea, so it is a recognizable and accessible way to take herbs.

A common way to make a cup of tea is to pour hot water over a tea bag and steep it for a few minutes. Although this is a pleasant way to enjoy herbal tea, making a medicinal-strength tea takes a little more time and effort. I recommend using loose herbs and not tea bags. They are often made from plastic and contain chemicals that can be harmful to the body. We do not want toxins in the medicina that we ingest!

The alchemy of tea is due to the interaction of the herbs and the water. As the herbs steep in the water, certain medicinal parts of the plant called phyto-chemicals are released. The longer the tea steeps, the more phytochemicals are absorbed into the water, thereby creating a stronger tea. When we make tea for medicine, we need time to let the herbs interact with the water so that we may create a powerful tea full of the medicinal properties of the plant.

There are different ways to make tea, depending on the different parts of the plants that are used. The two basic ways to make tea are called herbal infusions and herbal decoctions.

## Herbal Infusions

Herbal infusions are made by pouring water over herbs and allowing them to steep. Placing a tea bag in hot water is a kind of herbal infusion. However, to make a good, strong herbal infusion, we steep the herbs not just for a few minutes but for many hours. The best infusion will steep for about eight hours.

We use the more delicate parts of the plant, such as the leaves and flowers, to make herbal infusions. The temperature of the water used for herbal infusions is often hot, usually water that has just come to a boil. Other times, cold water works best. Cold-water infusions are good for herbs that have a lot of aromatic oils, such as yerba buena or manzanilla. Because heat can dissipate the volatile oils in the plant that give it flavor, by using cold water we can preserve the flavor and make a lovely, fragrant tea.

We also use cold-water infusions with mucilaginous plants, which have high amounts of starches called polysaccharides. The polysaccharides are what can give plants a slimy texture. The mucilage of a plant creates a moist coating of slime, which may sound gross but is actually very beneficial to the body. Plant mucilage can help lubricate dry or irritated mucous membranes of the respiratory or digestive tract, making it a useful remedy for sore throats, dry coughs, and certain kinds of digestive discomfort. A classic example of a mucilaginous plant that makes a good cold-water infusion is marshmallow root.

Some herbs can be used as either a hot- or cold-water infusion depending on what medicinal properties we hope to extract. A good example of such an herb is manzanilla. As a hot infusion steeped long enough, it will become bitter. However, as a cold infusion, it will retain its lovely fruity taste and be a pleasant-tasting beverage.

## Herbal Decoctions

Herbal decoctions are made by gently simmering herbs in hot water. Decoctions are best when working with the denser parts of plants, such as roots, seeds, and bark. It takes more energy to break down the cell walls of these tougher plant parts; therefore, we need higher temperatures to make herbal decoctions than for herbal infusions.

Herbs should be decocted for at least twenty minutes, yet you can get greater medicinal benefits by decocting your herbs for a much longer time. The longer herbs are decocted, the stronger the tea will be. When you decoct herbal tea for a long time, be sure to keep an eye on your decoction and add more water if necessary. I have definitely burned more than one pan by starting a decoction on my stove, then getting distracted and forgetting about it!

Herbs used in decoctions can often be decocted more than one time. First, strain off the liquid into a separate container. Next, add more water and simmer your herbs a second or even third time. The subsequent batches of tea will be less potent, but as long as you see color in the water and can taste the herbs, there is still medicine available.

# Tea-Making Instructions

## HERBAL INFUSION, HOT WATER

Parts used: Leaves, flowers

Amount: 1 tsp to 1 tbsp of dry herb or a small handful of fresh herb* per cup of water. The more herb you use, the stronger your tea will be.

Method: Add your herbs to a teapot or glass jar. Bring the water to a boil. Pour hot water over the herbs and cover. Steep for at least twenty minutes but ideally up to eight hours. Strain and drink.

## HERBAL INFUSION, COLD WATER

Parts used: Best for mucilaginous (slimy) plants such as marshmallow root, aloe, or comfrey, or for aromatic plants.

Amount: 1 tsp to 1 tbsp of dry herb or a handful of fresh herb per cup of water.

Method 1: Place herbs in a jar, cover with room-temperature water, and place in the refrigerator. Steep for eight hours. Strain and drink.

Method 2: This method works best with mucilaginous herbs. Place herbs in a small muslin bag and suspend it in cold water in a mason jar. Refrigerate eight hours. Strain the herbs and also use your hand to squeeze the slime from the bag into the water.

Additional note: Cold infusions are best drunk cold or at room temperature.

Some of my favorite herbs used for cold infusions are yerba buena, marshmallow root, rose, and manzanilla.

## HERBAL DECOCTION

Parts used: Roots, barks, seeds, twigs

Amount: 1 tsp to 1 tbsp of dry or fresh herb per cup of water. Some recipes for very strong decoctions recommend up to ½ oz of dried herb per cup of water.

---

* It is harder to get exact measurements when making tea from a fresh plant. I normally do not measure but flit around in my garden picking a little bit of this and a little bit of that to make my tea. If you are working with a plant that is safe and nontoxic, I recommend experimenting with different amounts of fresh plant material. More fresh plant material will make a stronger tea, so it depends also on your preference and your intention for making the tea.

Method: Put herbs and water in a stainless steel or ceramic saucepan and bring to a boil. Do not use aluminum pots. Gently simmer for at least twenty minutes and as long as several hours. Add more water if necessary to compensate for liquid lost by evaporation. Strain and drink. Herbs may be reused for a second or even third decoction.

Some of my favorite herbs to use for decoctions are burdock root, dandelion root, fennel, cinnamon, ginger, and astragalus.

# Drinking and Storing Herbal Tea

When drinking herbal tea for its medicinal properties, I usually recommend drinking one cup of tea one to three times a day. If you are making tea to help with sleep, normally a cup in the evening is sufficient. If a person is suffering from an acute health situation such as pain or a head cold, I also recommend drinking the medicinal tea throughout the day.

Once you have made your herbal infusion or decoction, strain out the plant material and refrigerate. Most herbal teas will store well in your refrigerator for three to five days.

You may drink your tea cold or gently reheat. When reheating your tea, do not use a microwave. Be careful not to boil your herbal infusions, as the high heat may change the taste and properties of the tea. You may sweeten your tea with honey, molasses, stevia, maple syrup, or other natural sweetener.

## HERBAL TEA RECIPES

Blending herbal tea is an art. As we become familiar with each herb's healing properties and each herb's flavor profile, we can combine them to create pleasant-tasting beverages. Here are some suggestions for recipes, but feel free to modify them and to create your own!

## INFUSIONS

### Nutritive Tea

1 part nettle
1 part oat straw
1 part red clover
1 part horsetail
1 part yerba buena

### Nerve Tonic Tea

2 parts oat straw
1 part scullcap
1 part lemon balm

### Soothing Lung Tea

1 part mullein
1 part marshmallow root
½ part licorice

## DECOCTIONS

### Digestive Tea

1 part ginger
1 part dandelion root
½ part fennel
¼ part cardamom

### Liver Support Tea

1 part dandelion root
1 part burdock root
1 part milk thistle seeds

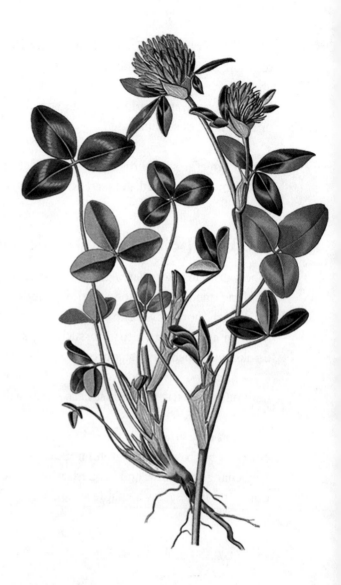

### Immune Support Tea

2 parts astragalus root
2 parts reishi mushroom
½ part ginger root
½ part licorice root

# Herbal Tinctures

Herbal tinctures are a popular and convenient way to take herbs, used by both Euro-American and Latinx herbal traditions. In tinctures, the medicinal properties of the plant are extracted into alcohol. Alcohol is a strong solvent and has the capacity to extract many phytochemicals from plants. Alcohol is also an excellent preservative, so tinctures can last for years, and I personally have tinctures in my apothecary that are over twenty-five years old and still viable.

The benefit of tinctures is their convenience. They can be taken straight from the bottle without any preparation. Tinctures are also easily transportable, so we can take our medicine throughout the day no matter where we are. The downside of tinctures is that they contain alcohol, which can make them unsuitable for people addicted to alcohol or with other sensitivities or liver problems.

If you are not strictly avoiding alcohol but don't like the taste, I recommend adding tincture to water or juice. Another option is to put the tincture in a mug and cover with boiling water so that the heat dissipates much of the alcohol. To remove more alcohol, I recommend adding the tincture to a small pot of water and gently boiling for a few minutes. Alternatives to alcohol-based tinctures include herbal glycerites, vinegars, or honeys.

## Tincture Making

Tinctures can be made from either fresh or dried plants. Fresh plants have more water content than dried and need a higher alcohol content to be preserved. When making tinctures from dried plants, we need to use more liquid because there is zero water content in the plant. In general, I prefer to use fresh plants for tinctures if I have access to them because fresh plants have more vitality and life force than dried plants.

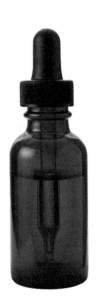

The first step to making tinctures is to break down your herb into the smallest size possible. The smaller-size pieces expose more surface area of the plant, which helps extract more of its phytochemicals. If I am working with the soft parts of a fresh plant, such as the leaves or flowers, I will tear them up with my hands or cut them with scissors or pruning shears. If I am working with a root, I will chop it up with pruning shears or a knife. Some people use blenders or grinders to process their plant material, but I prefer to work with my hands. For me, touching the plant is a way I interact with the medicine and get to know the plant.

The liquid medium in tinctures is called the *menstruum*. The percentage of alcohol in the menstruum varies from tincture to tincture. When you see 60 percent on a tincture bottle, this means that the menstruum is 60 percent alcohol.

There are several ways to make tinctures, some which involve precise weighing, measuring, and some computation. With the folk method, we don't need to be concerned with measuring but instead can use our creativity and intuition.

## The Folk Method

### INGREDIENTS AND MATERIALS

Herbs, either fresh or dried
80 proof (40%) or higher-proof alcohol (brandy, mezcal, rum, and the like)
Large bowl
Measuring cups
Glass jars
Labels

This method is best for dried herbs. If you use fresh herbs, I recommend dry-wilting the plants first before you tincture them. To dry-wilt a plant, just hang it or leave it out in a bowl for about twelve to twenty-four hours. As time passes, the plant loses its liquid, and the leaves will start to wilt. By wilting the plants, you decrease the amount of water that will exude into your menstruum from the plant, so that your final product has enough alcohol to prevent spoiling.

1. Cut, grind, or chop your herbs.
2. Loosely pack the herbs into a glass jar.
3. Pour hard alcohol of choice over the herbs and fill to the top of the jar.
4. Use a spoon to push the herbs down under the level of the alcohol.
5. If needed, place an unpolished stone on top of the herbs to keep them under the liquid.
6. Hold the jar and put your good intentions into the medicine.

7. Put the lid on the jar and label. Include on the label the date and the name of the herb.
8. Store in a place that is cool in temperature and out of direct light.
9. After one day, check to see whether all the herb material is covered by the alcohol. If not, add more.
10. After at least one moon cycle has passed, strain or press the herb. You can use cheesecloth or clean cotton. (I sometimes cut up old T-shirts or sheets.) Use a fine-meshed strainer to drain off the menstruum. Put the remaining plant material in a strainer lined with cheese cloth or cotton. Bundle up the herbs in the cloth and squeeze as hard as you can!
11. Bottle and label your tincture.
12. To preserve your tincture, store it in a dark amber bottle away from direct sunlight or heat.

# Herbal Cordials

Herbal cordials are alcohol-based herbal beverages. Tinctures are normally made of a single herb, whereas cordials are made of a combination of herbs and other ingredients.

Cordials are usually designed to be pleasant tasting and are enjoyed before, during, or after meals. Herbs are a key ingredient; some may include fruits and spices. Cordials are often sweetened to make them pleasing to drink.

## CORDIAL RECIPES

All cordials include fresh or dried herbs, alcohol (80 proof/40 percent or higher), and a natural sweetener of your choice. You can also add fresh or dried fruit.

### Basic Cordial Recipe, Maceration Method

1½ cups freshly packed herbs or ¾ cup dried herbs, spices, or flowers
2 cups mezcal, brandy, or other 80 proof (40%) alcohol
½ cup honey
Optional: 1 cup fresh fruit or ¼ cup dried fruit

1. Place herbs in a glass jar and cover with the alcohol.
2. Label your jar with the date and ingredients.
3. Shake well and let sit for one month.
4. After one month, strain liquid from the herbs.
5. Bottle the liquid and add honey to taste.

### Cordial Recipe, Decoction Method

This method works best with herbs that you would use for a decoction, such as seeds, roots, and bark.

1. Add ½ cup herbal seeds, bark, and/or roots to a stainless-steel pot.
2. Optional: 1 cup fresh or ½ cup dried fruit.
3. Cover with 2 cups water and simmer on low for about an hour, or until you have cooked off half the liquid.
4. Cool and strain off the liquid decoction.
5. Measure the amount of decoction.
6. Add 1 part alcohol per part of decoction. (For example, if you have 1 cup of decoction, add 1 cup of brandy as a preservative.)
7. Add ¼ cup honey per 1 cup of decoction.
8. Add more honey if desired.

### Elderberry Cordial Recipe

Elderberry cordial is a popular remedy for cold and flu season. It can be taken daily for prevention or used to address symptoms of cold and flu, including cough, sore throat, and congestion.

½ cup dried elderberries or 1 cup fresh
Brandy or other 80 proof (40%) alcohol
4 cups water
¼–½ cup honey
Optional: wild cherry bark, cinnamon, ginger, rose hips, star anise, mullein, thyme, sage

1.  Add elderberries and seeds, bark, and roots to a pan.
2.  Cover with 2 cups water and simmer.
3.  Add more water as needed if the level gets low.
4.  Decoct for at least 30 minutes and up to 2 hours. You want to decoct down to about half the amount of liquid.
5.  Turn off heat, add herbal flowers and leaves if you are using them.
6.  Steep one more hour.
7.  Strain and measure liquid.
8.  Add ¼ cup honey per 1 cup liquid.
9.  Add 1 part 80 proof (40%) alcohol to 1 part tea decoction.

Dosage: For adults as a preventive remedy, I recommend taking thirty to sixty drops daily of elderberry cordial. Increase the dosage to three to five times per day if you start feeling symptomatic, and continue to take this higher dose through the course of the cold. The dosage for children is much less and normally based on the child's weight, so consult an herbalist or trusted source when administering herbs to children. For children, drops can be mixed with water, juice, or honey.

### Digestive Delight Cordial Recipe

To support optimal digestive functioning and to be sipped as a beverage with meals. This recipe can be made using the decoction method.

> 1 tbsp cinnamon
> 1 tbsp cardamom
> 2 tbsp ginger
> ¼ cup dried dandelion root (or other herbal bitter, such as turmeric root, angelica root, or artichoke leaf)
> 2 cups mezcal, brandy, or other 80 proof (40%) alcohol

Dosage: For adults, take fifteen drops to ½ oz with meals.

### Heart-Mending Cordial Recipe

To help with grief, sadness, and heartbreak. This recipe can be made using the maceration method.

¼ cup hawthorn berries

¼ cup rose petals

Seeds of one fresh pomegranate

1 tbsp clove

1 tbsp cinnamon

2 cups mezcal, brandy, or alcohol of choice

Honey to taste

**Dosage:** For adults, take fifteen drops to ½ oz with meals.

## ENJOYING CORDIALS

Cordials are beverages meant to be sipped from tiny cups about the size of a shot glass. The amount consumed varies anywhere from ⅛ tsp to 1 oz. To decrease the alcohol taste, mix your cordial with water. To make a refreshing drink, mix the cordial with bubbly water.

# Flower Essences

Modern flower essence therapy was developed by an English man named Edward Bach in the early 1900s and has been adopted by people worldwide. Flower essences support emotional, mental, and spiritual health, and are excellent remedies to support our healing journey and our work with los aires.[*]

Flower essences are a form of energetic medicine made from fresh blooming flowers. Each essence contains the flower's vibrational imprint, which carries its unique qualities and healing properties.

When we take a flower essence, our entire being is bathed with the vibration of the color, shape, and aroma of that flower. The flower essence attunes us to the vibrations of Tonantzin, which helps harmonize our own energy. As our energy is harmonized, what is challenging us, such as difficult emotions or behaviors, nat-

---

[*] Flower essences can help to harmonize all of the thirteen aires, which will be discussed in more depth in chapter 11.

urally begin to shift and dissolve. I regularly use flower essences for myself and recommend them to all my clients, students, friends, and family. Flower essences work great for children, animals, and plants as well. My cats are regularly (albeit reluctantly) dosed with flower essences.

## Making Flower Essences

A flower essence is basically a flower tea made of the blossoms infused into water in full sunlight. After we make our flower tea, it is diluted down to a homeopathic level and preserved. For me, making flower essences is both a ritual and a meditation with the plant and flower. I take time to quiet my mind, be still, and sit with the plant. I closely observe the plant and patiently wait and listen to its messages for me.

### INGREDIENTS AND MATERIALS

Fresh flowers in full bloom (from a living plant in the earth)
Glass bowl or chalice
Water
80 proof (40%) alcohol or vinegar
Measuring cup
Strainer
Funnel
Small glass jar
Amber bottles to store finished essence
Labels

1. Decide which flower to work with and choose a flower that is vital and in full bloom. Be mindful to choose a flower that is abundant; leave plenty for the animals and pollinators.
2. Clean the glass vessel and fill it with water.
3. Offer prayers; make an offering to the plant, asking permission to pick a few of its flowers. Once I have selected the plant I will work with, I first prepare my space. I like to create a small outdoor altar with stones or other objects from the nature around me.

4.  Choose a few twigs or rocks from nearby and use them to gently pick the blossoms. To keep the energy of the flower uncontaminated, do not touch the flowers with your hands. Catch the blossoms in the bowl of water. Alternatively, flower essences can be made without picking the flower. This is called a living flower essence. This is the best method when working with rare or endangered flowers or when there is not an abundance of flowers to pick. Some people prefer this method for all flower essences, because it does not disrupt the life force of the flower. To make a living flower essence, gently lean the flower into the water. Sometimes the bowl of water needs to be elevated to reach the plant, or we need to use sticks or even string to help the flower stay in the water. If it is impossible to get the flower into the water, another option is to place the bowl of water at the base of the flower and invite the spirit of the flower into the water.

5.  Let the flower remain in the water and sunlight for some time, usually at least three hours, although I have made essences in much less time. Sometimes I like to keep my essences out from sunrise to sunset. Listen to your own intuition and listen to what the plant guides you to do. The flower water is ready when it looks sparkly and bubbly. Sometimes the bowl will attract insects, which is OK; it just means that the essence has a little ant or spider medicine as well.

6.  When your flower water is finished, strain this "mother essence" into a small glass jar or bottle. To preserve the mother essence, add alcohol or vinegar at about a 2:1 ratio to the flower water. Immediately label your bottle with the words "mother essence" and add the date, name of the plant, and location where it was made.*

7.  Dilute the mother essence to make the stock essence, which I like to call the "daughter" or "child" essence. First fill a 1 oz amber bottle with brandy or vinegar. Shake the mother essence well. Add a few drops of the mother essence to the amber bottle. Flower essences that are sold in stores are usually stock essences; you can take flower essences straight from the stock bottles.

---

* A way to learn more about the flower essence is to take a little sip of the mother water (see step 6). Drinking the mother water "proves" the remedy, which means it can bring forth the conditions that it treats. Be careful, because this can activate unpleasant feelings. Normally this state of proving the remedy only lasts for about twenty minutes, but it can be quite uncomfortable. Also, if you are working with a toxic plant, never ingest the mother water undiluted.

8.	(Optional) Create a dosage bottle by adding four drops of the stock essence into a tincture or into a base of brandy or vinegar. Dosage bottles allow us to blend flower essences together or to add them to herbal tinctures.

## Using Flower Essences

Flower essences are very versatile, and there are many ways to incorporate them into our daily lives. Here are some suggestions on how to use flower essences:

- Shake well! Shaking helps activate the energy of the flower essence.
- Take four drops four times per day of the stock or dosage bottle.
- Add four drops of essence to a mister bottle to use as a spray.
- Apply drops topically or add to creams, lotions, or baths.
- For children, add one to four drops of a flower essence to juice or water. For animals, add one to four drops to their food or drinking water. For diseased or injured plants, add flower essences to the water you give them.

To amplify the effects of flower essences, take them more frequently. Each time we take the essence, we are infusing ourselves with its energies, so by increasing the frequency we are intensifying the effects. Flower essences are gentle and safe, but sometimes can elicit strong reactions. As they move our energies, they may activate healing opportunities or healing crises. In other words, they can stir up our shit. When this happens, I recommend that folks take their formula less often. Another strategy is to take the essence more often, so that we move through our healing process more quickly. When working with clients, I always advise them to contact me if they feel as though the essences have triggered a healing crisis. Sometime folks need to stop taking their essences until they feel more settled.

## Enhancing Flower Essence Work

Flower essences will work well on their own without much effort on our part. However, we can enhance their effects by bringing our intention and focus to the process. Here are some strategies that I recommend for enhancing their effect:

- Set your intention for the medicine you are creating for yourself.
- Write down the essences you are taking and how they work.
- Keep a journal of your process. Pay attention to how the theme of the flower essence is moving through your life.
- Take your flower essences before mediation or prayer.
- Take your flower essences before going to sleep at night.
- Take your essence regularly for at least one moon cycle. When you've finished the bottle, take time to journal and reflect on your process.

Some essences we need for a month; some we need for a lifetime. Essences can support us in acute situations and when working with long-standing core issues.

# Medicine-Making Journals

Each of us brings our creativity, passion, and inspiration to our medicine making. More than once, I have invented something wonderful but am unable to replicate it because I did not take notes. I have found it helpful to keep a journal for my medicine making. I write down my recipes (when I remember) so that I am able to duplicate them in the future. I have kept one notebook for decades; it contains the earliest prototypes of some of my recipes, which eventually became my products.

May the medicina you make be powerful, healing, and beneficial to you and your loved ones! May your process be joyous and help you to deepen your relationship to your plant allies!

# SPOTLIGHT

# Batul True Heart
## (they/them/theirs/aapo)

> "I came into Curanderismo for personal survival. I wouldn't be here without it. The biggest blessing [of walking with ancestral medicine] has been healing fragmentation and standing in wholeness."

Batul True Heart is queer, two-spirit, and of Yo'eme (Yaqui), Mexican, Panamanian American (Indigenous, African, Spanish), and English descent. They were born on Tongva land, raised on Pomo land, and currently live in Huchiun/Oakland.

I met Batul at the Two-Spirit Powwow in San Francisco. A mutual friend introduced us because she knew of our shared interest in ancestral medicine. We connected instantly, and Batul became my student, friend, colleague, and eventually a core teacher in the Curanderx Toolkit class. Fiercely dedicated to healing, Batul is a gifted teacher, herbalist and limpiadore, and death doula, and creator of the herbal business Maaso Medicina: Medicine for Ancestral, Generational, and Personal Pain. Through Maaso Medicina, Batul created a flower essence line to address each of the thirteen aires.

## BATUL TRUE HEART SPEAKS:

My Panamanian bisabuela, Pastora Cornejo, read tarot cards, wrote spells, and put marijuana in alcohol for arthritis. She never let me go outside with my hair wet, always made sure I had socks on, made traditional foods like Panamanian-style arroz con pollo, and nursed injured and abandoned baby deer back to life. I now know these practices are curanderismo.

Colonialism tore my Yo'eme family apart, but I now know that my Yaqui bisabuela, Virginia Michicho Sanchez, *also* put marijuana in alcohol for joints, had a cactus garden, made the best handmade tortillas in Arizona, and spoke our Yaqui language. (It's only been lost for two generations, and now I'm bringing it back!!)

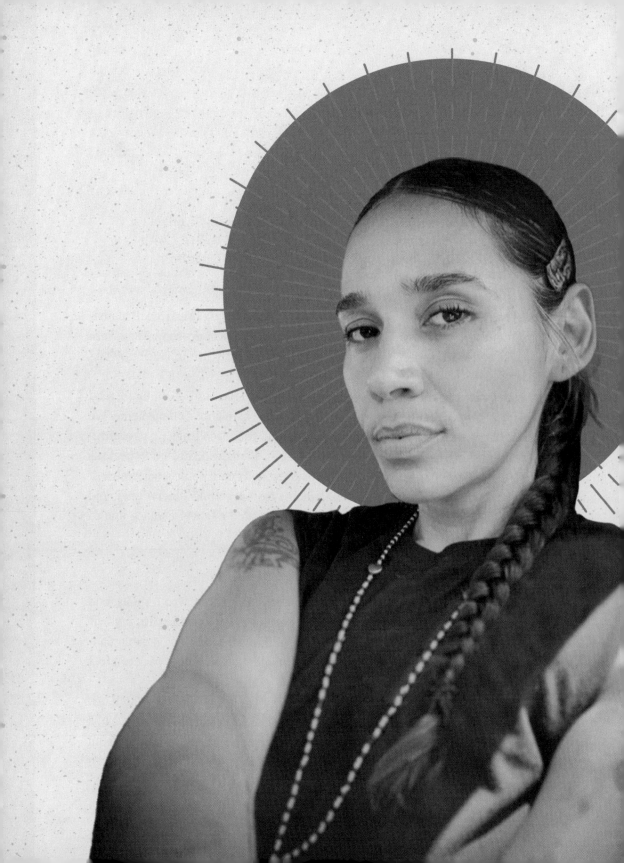

Because of settler colonial assimilation, I did not grow up around my traditional Yaqui ancestral ways. I only had my baby moccasins and my baby huaraches to remind me of my roots. Instead, I was a mixed Yaqui child living in and around a white, colonial, Christian, homophobic, and patriarchal experience. Still, though, I've always been Yo'eme, through and through.

Curanderismo came into my life after I had a peyote ceremony for myself. I made a prayer in front of the medicine, the fire, and my community, to "be who I truly am." This prayer was a plea to find wholeness within myself after feeling so deeply fragmented because of colonialism. Seven weeks later, I met Atava, and she invited me to attend the Curanderx Toolkit class. Soon after that, I met Estela Román and have received both healing and mentoring from her. I've been deeply dedicated to the path ever since.

"Maaso Medicina is also the medicine I bring through my words and messages (through speaking, writing, photos), which is one of *the* medicines that comes directly from my Yaqui ancestors. Our name means "Those who speak as loud as the Yaqui River" or "Those who talk with Authority." I am a speaker. This is one way I move energy. I also hold space for people and hold people through the dying process.

Challenges are a necessary part of the path. I'd say the biggest challenges I've faced are the deep remnants of colonialism that have kept me feeling inadequate, unworthy, guilty, and like a fraud. Those same difficulties (aires), though, once faced and felt through, only make me more CHINGONX [badass].

To me, it doesn't matter whether you grew up with this medicine or not. It's a wonderful thing when a child is raised with Indigenous roots intact and when medicine and healing are taught throughout childhood, but the truth is that hardly any of us (who are Native/Indigenous), at this point, got that. Many of us cherish the fragments of the medicine that were kept alive, but many of us have not had consistency with the medicine. And this, to me, is the key. This medicine wants to be in constant relationship with us. Our healing work can only deepen through our dedication and through knowing what a great responsibility and privilege it is to know *and* walk with the traditional medicine of our ancestors.

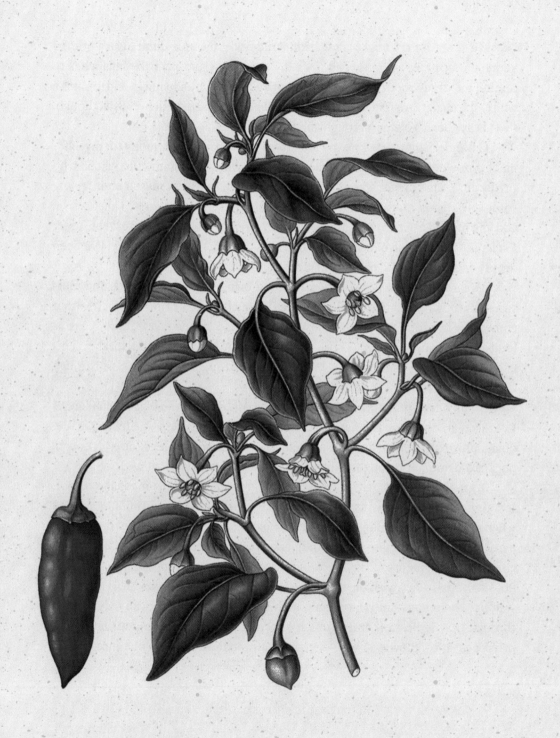

# CHAPTER 9

# Nourishment: Herbal Tonics and Food as Medicine

Our opportunity to interact with herbal medicine expands beyond taking tinctures, teas, or cordials. Each day, we can receive the healing benefits of herbs by incorporating them into our meals as food and spices. Herbal medicine offers us something that pharmaceutical drugs do not, which is the plants' ability to nourish the cells, tissues, and organs of our bodies. As I've mentioned elsewhere, herbs are made up of dozens of molecules called phytochemicals. When we ingest herbs, these phytochemicals mingle with the cells in our bodies and create optimal cellular environments to promote health and prevent disease. In other words, by supporting the optimal functioning of our body's cells, tissues, and organs, herbal medicine can be an excellent form of preventive medicine. When we build relationship with plants, every day, every meal is an opportunity to receive their blessings.

## Herbal Tonics

In herbal medicine, we have a category of herbs called herbal tonics. Herbal tonics are herbs that support the healthy functioning of the body's tissues, organs, and cells. They help optimize the body's processes, such as digestion, absorption of nutrients, and detoxification. Herbal tonics often have high nutritional value and are an easy way to incorporate nutrient-dense foods into our diets.

Herbal tonics are safe for most people to take on a long-term basis and generally have few contraindications. By incorporating herbal tonics into our daily lives, we can boost our energy, increase our sense of well-being, and prevent illness.

Different herbal tonics have affinity for different organs and organ systems of the body. For example, raspberry leaf is a well-known tonic for the womb.

Hawthorn is a tonic for the heart and the cardiovascular system. Some herbal tonics, such as nettles, work in a more general way by nourishing many organ systems of the body and by providing vitamins and minerals and supporting the body in its natural processes of elimination.

We may take our herbal tonics in any form that we regularly consume our herbal medicine. This includes drinking herbal tea or taking herbal tinctures or capsules. Herbal tonics are also great to incorporate into meals as vinegars, oils, or herbal sprinkles. Some tonic herbs, such as burdock root, are delicious to eat as food. Tonantzin has blessed us with hundreds of herbal tonics, and here I will share two of my favorite traditional remedies.

## Ortiga/Stinging Nettle

*Urtica dioica*

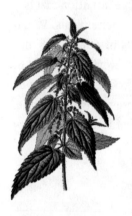

Stinging nettle is native to North Africa, Europe, and Central Asia and has naturalized in many regions of the world, including California and northern Mexico. Nettles grow wild in natural spaces across California, and they can be easily cultivated in Huchiun/Bay Area gardens. They can be propagated from seeds or root division and prefer rich, moist soil and full to partial shade.[1] This plant is named stinging nettle because it has fine hairs on its stalks and leaves that can cause pain, redness, and swelling when in contact with skin.

Stinging nettle is a plant packed with vitamins and minerals. I like to say that consuming nettles is like taking a daily multivitamin. They are high in calcium, iron, magnesium, potassium, phosphorus, vitamin A, B vitamins, and vitamin K.[2] Many of my students report that regularly taking nettles gives them more energy. Nettles can improve the health of skin, hair, bones, and joints. People who consume nettles on a daily basis will notice that their skin begins to glow, and their hair becomes thicker and glossier.

Nettles are high in calcium, and I recommend nettles for people who are concerned about losing bone density. They are an excellent herbal ally to support elders who are dealing with osteoporosis. To receive the maximum amount of calcium and other minerals from nettles, I recommend making a nettle vinegar.

The acidity of vinegar helps extract the calcium and other minerals from the plant. Nettles also have good amounts of iron and can be useful for people dealing with anemia.

Nettles have many other medicinal properties. They help with skin conditions, seasonal allergies, and arthritis. They help the body's organs detoxify, and decrease inflammation in the body. The sting of nettles is a legendary remedy to relieve pain and stiffness in joints. The therapeutic practice of flogging the body with nettles is called urtification and has been used for thousands of years by cultures around the world. Doña Enriqueta recommends applying fresh nettles to the back of the knees "para los nervios," or to relieve stress and anxiety.[3]

On my herb walks, I usually ask if anyone in the group is experiencing physical pain and ask for someone to volunteer themselves for a nettle treatment. Usually we have one brave volunteer who agrees to be gently flogged with nettles on their painful body part. I always share that this treatment is done with love and prayers for the relief of their pain. The rest of the class huddles around the volunteer and watches closely as red welts appear in the area of skin that has been stung. The volunteer reports an initial stinging and burning sensation, which usually is followed in ten to fifteen minutes by a significant decrease of their pain.

# Avena/Wild Oat

*Avena sativa*

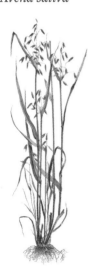

Wild oat, also called oatstraw, is native to Europe but has naturalized in California. It loves growing on sunny slopes and meadows, and reseeds itself each year. Wild oat is related to the cultivated oats that are grown for food.

With their long, cylindrical stalks and hanging seed pods, oats are fairly easy to identify. The seed pods look like dangling earrings. In the spring, the oat stalks are bright green, but by the end of summer, they dry out and turn a golden color. Fields of oats swaying and dancing with the wind can be found across many open meadows around Huchiun/the Bay Area. Both the seed pods and the stalks or straw of oats can be used for medicine. The seed tops are best harvested when they are fresh and milky and should be used that same day.

Milky oat tops are an excellent tonic for both the nerves and the adrenal glands. Oats are high in both calcium and magnesium, which are essential nutrients for the nervous system. They are a great herbal ally to support people dealing with chronic stress. Oats can help soothe frayed nerves and mitigate the effects of stress in our bodies, including jumpiness, anxiety, and insomnia. As a nervous system tonic, oats support our bodies to recover when we feel exhausted and depleted from stress. Oats can bring a sense of feeling calm, grounded, and nourished.

## Food as Medicine

Food is an essential part of nuestra medicina. Many of our traditional foods, such as corn, beans, squash, and chilis, provide us with all the nutrients we need for good health. The spices used to flavor our foods, such as oregano, rosemary, basil, chili, cumin, and cilantro, all have healing properties. When we add spices and herbs to our food, we receive the double benefit of something that tastes delicious and also is infused with essential nutrients. There are countless ways to incorporate herbs into cooking.

In this chapter, I will discuss the healing properties of a few ingredients commonly used in Mexican cuisine. The list of herbs used in traditional Mexican cuisine is extensive and varies regionally, so I am choosing to write about a few that are most accessible and affordable. These herbs are available in most grocery stores and can be grown easily in most California climates. I also share a few of my favorite recipes for incorporating herbal medicine into food.

# Orégano/Oregano

At least three different plants in Mexican curanderismo share the same common name "oregano."* All have medicinal benefits and are often used interchangeably, although they are different species of plants from different parts of the world. This can cause confusion for herbalists and other people using these plants. For clarity, I will explain a little about each kind of oregano.

## MEDITERRANEAN OREGANO
*Origanum vulgare*\*\*

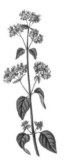

Mediterranean oregano originated in Greece, and the word *oregano* can be translated from Greek to mean "joy of the mountain." This hardy perennial shrub has small, oval-shaped leaves and is a member of the mint or Lamiaceae plant family. Oregano was a popular spice and medicine in Europe in the Middle Ages, used for respiratory infections, digestive troubles, toothaches, convulsions, dropsy, wounds, and snake bites.

Oregano became popular in North America after World War II when soldiers who had been stationed in Italy brought it back home after the war.[4] In Mexico, Mediterranean oregano has been thoroughly incorporated as both a food and a medicine. Oregano has strong antiviral properties and as a medicinal herb is used for sore throats, cough, colds, and other respiratory infections. Doña Enriqueta recommends combining oregano with cinnamon to treat fever and chest pain from respiratory infections. She also recommends using oregano for menstrual cramps and as a postpartum aid.[5] Oregano supports the digestive system and can be used for stomachaches, cramping, gas, and intestinal infections.

---

\* Often the same common name will be shared by more than one plant. The "common name" is the name used by local people. One plant may have many different common names depending on the culture, language, or geographical area it comes from. This can be very confusing! I have found it helpful to learn the or scientific binomial (Latin names) of each plant. I resisted learning the scientific names for years because it felt like a colonial way of identifying plants. However, I have grown to embrace identifying plants by both their common and scientific names. This way I can understand exactly which plant is being talking about. It also helps to know scientific names for plants when working across languages and cultures.

\*\* To make matters more confusing, sometimes *Origanum vulgare* is referred to as marjoram.

*Origanum vulgare* is easy to grow in many climates. It prefers full sun, is drought tolerant, and can be cultivated from seeds or cuttings. It is also an easy plant to grow in pots. I love to have fresh oregano available to add to meals I am cooking.

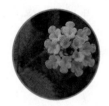

### ORÉGANO/MEXICAN OREGANO/DESERT OREGANO/AHUIYAXIHUITL
*Lippia graveolens* (shown)
*Lippia wrightii*
*Lippia* spp

Mexican oregano belongs to the vervain or Verbenaceae plant family. It is a small desert shrub with oval-shaped leaves that are larger and thicker than *Origanum vulgare*. Its native habitat includes the US Southwest, Mexico, and Central America and had been used for centuries before European contact.[6] Because it is native to warmer climates, it enjoys sun and is drought tolerant, but can't handle freezing temperatures. It can be propagated through seeds and cuttings.[7] It is used traditionally to treat colds, fever, broken bones, and ailments of the digestive tract.[8]

Mexican oregano is aromatic and carminative, which means it stimulates and supports digestion. It helps with gas, bloating, and intestinal infections and parasites. Like Mediterranean oregano, it also can be used to treat menstrual cramps, earaches, toothaches, colds, cough, and fever.[9]

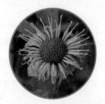

### ORÉGANO DE LA SIERRA/ORÉGANO DEL CAMPO/WILD OREGANO/BEE BALM
*Monarda* spp

*Monarda* grows across the American continent and many parts of Mexico and is a lovely perennial plant in the mint family. Its cheerful flowers, which range in color from pale pink to blue and purple, are a favorite of many pollinators, including bees, butterflies, and moths. The scent of *Monarda* is similar to Mediterranean oregano, but its flavor tends to be stronger and more pungent. *Monarda* can be propagated with seeds or root division, and it prefers to grow in full sun or partial shade.[10]

*Monarda* species plants are important traditional medicines used by many Indigenous people across Turtle Island. In Mexican and Mexican American herbalism, it is cherished as a remedy for colds, coughs, fevers, sore throats, and other issues of the respiratory tract. Like the other oreganos, it is carminative and aromatic, and benefits digestion.

## RECOMMENDATIONS FOR USE OF ALL KINDS OF OREGANO

Add fresh or dried herb to savory foods, soup stock, spice sprinkles, and herbal oils and vinegars. Can be tinctured and also makes a tasty tea.

## CONTRAINDICATIONS

All three plants stimulate uterine contractions, so should be avoided in pregnancy.

# Epazote/Wormseed/Epazotl
*Dysphania ambrosioides*

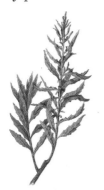

Epazote is native to Mexico and the Southwest, where it is treasured as both a culinary and medicinal herb. The name epazote comes from the Nahuatl word *epazotl*, which translates to "skunk odor." Its remarkable odor, which to me smells like gasoline, makes it easy to identify. Epazote grows easily from seeds, likes full sun, and can tolerate both heat and dry conditions. In colder climates, it acts as an annual, but will continue to grow through the winter in warmer climates.[11]

Epazote has been used traditionally to treat worms and other parasites and is a digestive remedy to treat intestinal infections, diarrhea, gas, and bloating. It is used topically as a poultice for fungal infections, warts, wounds, and insect bites. Epazote is used to relieve menstrual cramps and to accelerate contractions during childbirth, and in the temescal for postpartum treatments. It also is used in limpias to relieve susto, espanto, and other mal aires.[12] Epazote is commonly used in Mexican cooking to flavor food and also to support digestion. Adding epazote to a pot of beans will help us more easily digest the beans (which means less bloating and gas!).

## SUGGESTIONS FOR USE

Add to beans, soups, stews, moles, salsas, eggs, vegetables, and meat dishes. Drink as a tea, add to vinegar, or add to an herbal sprinkle.

## CONTRAINDICATIONS

Epazote is a strong medicine and should be used with caution. Large quantities can cause nausea and induce vomiting. Because epazote stimulates the uterus, it should be avoided in pregnancy.

# Chile/Chili Pepper/Chilli

*Capsicum* spp

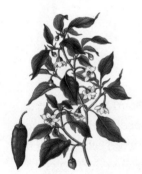

Chile, which has been cultivated in Mexico for thousands of years, is a staple of Mexican cuisine and an essential part of Mexican culture. The common names in English (chili) and Spanish (chile) are both derived from the Nahuatl word for the plant, *chilli*. The first chili peppers originated in South America (either in Brazil or Bolivia) and were spread across the American continents with the help of birds.

The first people to cultivate chile were in ancient Mexico, at least six thousand years ago.[13] The species of chili most cultivated was *Capsicum annuum*, whose varieties include cayenne, jalapeño, serrano, and New Mexican green and red chilis. Today the greatest biodiversity of *Capsicum* varieties can be found in Mexico. Chili loves growing in rich soil; it prefers heat and full sun and is easily propagated by seeds.

Chile is beloved as a food for its flavor and heat, and it is also a true panacea of herbal medicine. Chile has been used traditionally to help with arthritis, digestion, parasites, and ailments of the respiratory tract. The spiciness of chile activates the flow of mucous and helps clear congestion in the sinuses and bronchioles—anyone who has eaten hot salsa has experienced this! Chile helps warm the body and stimulate circulation. The primary phytochemical in the *Capsicum* species is called capsaicin, which has been found in studies to help decrease pain. To treat pain, ingest chile internally as a food or medicine or use it topically as a poultice, oil, salve, or liniment. Capsaicin also has been found in studies to reduce both blood sugar and blood cholesterol levels.

## SUGGESTIONS FOR USE

In addition to its culinary use as a spice, chile may be added to herbal vinegars (see the Fuego recipe later in this chapter), broths, infused oils, and tinctures. Topically chile can be added to oils, salves, and liniments. Be careful not to get chile in the eyes or other mucous membranes.

## CONTRAINDICATIONS

May burn the skin or mucous membranes. Avoid in cases of excess stomach acid or reflux. Chile stimulates circulation and thins the blood, so avoid during surgeries, and use with caution when taking blood-thinning medications.

# Cilantro/Coriander

*Coriandrum sativum*

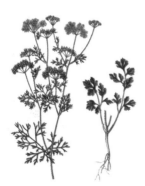

Although it is not a native to Mexico, cilantro has become a key ingredient in many Mexican dishes today. Cilantro, which originates from North Africa, Southeast Asia, and Southern Europe, is actually the same plant as the spice called coriander. The name cilantro refers to the fresh leaves, whereas coriander refers to the dried seeds. Cilantro can be easily grown from seeds and can grow well in pots. It prefers part shade and cooler temperatures. In the heat, it will bolt (go to seed) quickly.

Coriander seeds are carminative, which means they support healthy digestive functioning. A tea from the seeds is helpful for stomachaches, colic, digestive cramps, and gas. Coriander is mildly sedating, and a strong tea will help with sleep. The seeds have also been used traditionally as mouthwash for sore and inflamed gums, or as a gargle for a sore throat.

Cilantro leaves are highly nutritious and packed with antioxidants, vitamins, and minerals, including iron and magnesium. Freshly chopped leaves make a delicious addition to salsas, soups, and salads. Doña Enriqueta recommends eating cilantro in a salad with onion for people who feel weak or who are recuperating from a cold and need to strengthen their lungs, and recommends eating cilantro in caldo de res (beef soup) to build the blood.[14] One of cilantro's magical powers is its ability to help the body clear out toxins from the blood. Cilantro helps with chelation of heavy metals, which means it helps bind to such metals as lead and mercury so that they may be excreted out through the urine.[15] Although many people love cilantro, certain people have a particular gene that makes them dislike its taste.

## SUGGESTIONS FOR USE

Add fresh cilantro to salsa, pesto, salads, soups, smoothies, and vinegars or as a garnish for meals. Coriander seeds can be used as a spice or decocted and drunk as a tea.

## CONTRAINDICATIONS

Some people have an allergic reaction to cilantro when it is ingested or handled topically.

# Ajo/Garlic

*Allium sativum*

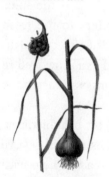

Garlic originated in Central Asia and has been used as a medicinal plant for over five thousand years. It can be easily propagated in most climates by planting its bulbs in the fall so that its roots can grow through the winter. Garlic is used to treat colds, flu, viruses, bronchitis, cough, digestive problems, hypertension, high cholesterol, arteriosclerosis, and cancer, and is used topically as an antibiotic to treat wounds.

Garlic is rich in sulfur compounds, which are beneficial to the immune system. Numerous scientific studies have correlated the consumption of garlic with decreased risk of different types of cancer, including gastric, colon, and prostate cancer.[16] Garlic stimulates immune cells, such as lymphocytes and macrophages, which protect the body against viruses, bacteria, and parasites.[17] These sulfur compounds in garlic have a special affinity for the respiratory system. When we ingest garlic, these compounds are excreted into the bloodstream and are eliminated through the lungs. We breathe out garlic compounds, creating the infamous garlic breath. Garlic breath is a good sign! It tells us that the garlic compounds are present in the respiratory system. They go directly to the tissue in our lungs, bronchioles, and throat to help fight infections, such as colds or bronchitis.

## SUGGESTIONS FOR USE

Add garlic to dishes as a spice, vinegar, honey, infused oil, or pesto. Garlic is most potent when eaten raw. To optimize its cancer-fighting effects, cut raw garlic and let it sit about ten minutes before cooking.

## CONTRAINDICATIONS

Some people's digestive systems are irritated by garlic. Do not take if you are experiencing chronic gastrointestinal inflammation. May be present in breast milk, so avoid when breastfeeding. Garlic thins the blood, so don't use it if undergoing surgery. Consult with an herbalist about using garlic if you're taking blood-thinning medications.

# Cebolla/Onion

*Allium cepa*
*Allium glandulosum*

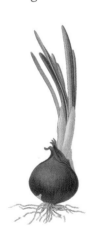

For more than six thousand years, onions have been used as a food and medicine by ancient cultures in Africa, Asia, Mesopotamia, and Europe. The common culinary yellow onion, *Allium cepa*, originated in Central Asia, but has been cultivated all around the world. Different varieties of wild onion are native to many continents, including the Americas. *Allium glandulosum*, called xonacatl in Nahuatl, was commonly used across Central Mexico before European contact. Onions are cold tolerant and are best grown from bulbs in either spring or fall.[18]

Onions' medicinal properties are similar to garlic.

Onions benefit the digestive, immune, cardiovascular, and respiratory systems. They are high in fiber as well as the prebiotic inulin, which are both beneficial to the microbiome of the digestive tract. Traditionally onions have been used to treat colds, flu, cough, bronchitis, and high blood pressure. Onions are high in vitamins, minerals, and the bioflavonoid quercetin. Quercetin is a powerful antioxidant that plays an important role in heart health and also protects cells against oxidative damage. Red onions contain more quercetin than other varieties of onion. Quercetin is most concentrated in the onion peel and in the top three layers of the onion, and is most bioavailable in raw onions.[19] Scientific research has found that onions, like garlic, have cancer-fighting properties.[20]

Onions can be used topically as a poultice and are especially helpful for breaking up congestion in the lungs and respiratory tract. My cousin, who is a frontline nurse working with patients with COVID-19, unfortunately contracted the coronavirus at work. While my cousin was in quarantine and couldn't go out to the store to buy medicine, I offered suggestions for herbal support, starting by asking whether she had any onions in her kitchen. She replied yes, and I recommended that she make an onion poultice for her chest. She made the poultice and reported back that it made a huge difference in clearing the congestion in her lungs.

Onions are safe for most people to ingest. However, they do have blood-thinning effects, so people on blood-thinning medications or undergoing surgery should be careful and avoid large amounts of onion. Some people who are sensitive to onions may experience gas and bloating when ingesting them.

## SUGGESTIONS FOR USE

Add to savory dishes. Eat raw in salsa and on salads, or sprinkle raw onion on soups or other hot dishes. Onion can be used as an herbal vinegar, honey, or infused oil.

## RECIPES

### HERBAL-INFUSED BROTHS

One of my favorite ways to make food my medicine is by making medicinal broths. As I stand in my kitchen stirring a big pot of soup, watching the vegetables and herbs swirl in the hot water, I feel my ancestors close to me. For me, making broth is ancestral alchemy. I feel connected to the long line of women who learned how to survive in times of hardship by making soup from whatever they could forage from their gardens or nearby fields, or whatever scraps of vegetables were left in the pantry. In the wintertime, I make a big batch of broth weekly and drink a cup every day. Any herb can be added to soup stocks, depending on the flavors you are seeking and what ingredients you have available on hand.

I like to save my vegetable scraps for my stock. I keep them in a bag in my freezer and take them out when needed. I also save the leftover herb material from tincture or vinegar making (such as Fuego cider) to add to the stock. Vegans and vegetarians can make delicious and nutritious stocks entirely from plants. For people who eat meat, adding bones from poultry, fish, lamb, beef, pork, or wild game will add extra nutrients to your stock, including minerals such as calcium, magnesium, and phosphorus, as well as amino acids and collagen.

Many traditional Mexican recipes, such as posole and menudo, are based on slow-cooked broths made of herbs, vegetables, bones, and meat. Herbal broths are lovely to share with others to support their healing. After I underwent surgery for cancer, my friends brought me food to support my recovery. Some of the most healing and nourishing foods I received were soups and broths. I could feel my cells dancing with each sip!

### Plant-Powered Broth

4 quarts water
1 onion
2–4 cloves garlic
2 carrots
2 celery stalks
2–4 kale ribs (or other vegetable stalks, such as collards, broccoli, or chard)

1 piece of kombu (about 6–8 inches) or other seaweed

2 slices of reishi mushroom (about 4 inches long)

¼ cup dried nettles (1 cup fresh)

¼ cup dried burdock root (1 cup fresh)

4-inch slice ginger root

4-inch slice turmeric root

Optional: any other vegetable scraps, edible or medicinal mushrooms, or herbs

1. Add all ingredients to a large soup pot. Cover with water.
2. Bring to a boil and simmer on low for at least two hours. Alternatively, you may cook in a crock pot or pressure cooker.
3. Strain. Add salt, pepper, and/or lemon to taste. May be served with fresh parsley, cilantro, or other fresh greens. Refrigerate (up to three days) or freeze (up to three months).

### Herbal-Infused Bone Broth

4 quarts water

2–3 lbs. bones (chicken, beef, pork, lamb, fish, or wild game)*

2 tbsp vinegar

1 onion

1–2 carrots

1–2 celery stalks

2–3 cloves garlic

1 generous pinch of fresh or dried rosemary, thyme, oregano, and/or sage

Optional: reishi or other medicinal mushroom, nettles, burdock, seaweed, turmeric, or any other herb

*For richer flavor, roast bones in the oven at 350 degrees until brown.

1. Add bones to pot and cover with water.
2. Add the vinegar. The acid in the vinegar helps break down the bones and make their minerals more bioavailable. Allow it to sit for twenty minutes.

3. Add the rest of the ingredients, bring to a boil, cover and cook on low for twelve to thirty-six hours on the stove or in a slow cooker. If cooking on the stove top, check regularly to make sure there's enough liquid.

## HERBAL VINEGARS

A great way to incorporate herbs into your cooking is to make a medicinal vinegar. Vinegar extracts medicinal properties from plants and is a common nonalcoholic base for herbal medicines. The acidic nature of vinegar is particularly helpful for extracting calcium, iron, potassium, magnesium, and other minerals from plants. Many modern diets are deficient in minerals, so consuming herbal vinegars is a good way to boost the mineral content in our diets. Minerals are essential for our health, and mineral deficiencies are linked to many diseases. Vinegar is also a good preservative, and herbal vinegars usually have a shelf life of at least a year.

Herbal vinegars can be used in any recipe that calls for vinegar. I like to use mine in salad dressings or to dress cooked veggies and greens. Herbal vinegars can be taken straight or added to water and sipped as a beverage. Either fresh or dried herbs can be used to infuse vinegars.

### Basic Herbal Vinegar Recipe

Glass jar with lid
1 cup chopped fresh herbs or ¼ cup dried herbs
2 cups vinegar of your choice (apple cider, balsamic, rice vinegar, wine vinegar, and so on)

1. Add herbs to jar.
2. Cover herbs with vinegar. Make sure all herbs are below the liquid. Add more vinegar if needed.
3. Place plastic wrap or a plastic bag on top of the jar. This keeps the metal lid from rusting.
4. Cover with the lid (on top of the plastic).
5. Label your jar with the date and ingredients.
6. Shake well and put your love into your medicine.
7. Store out of direct light and heat for one moon cycle. Shake regularly.

8. Strain after one moon cycle. Pour liquid into glass bottles.
9. Add honey to taste if desired.

### High-Mineral Vinegar

1 cup fresh or ¼ cup dried nettles, wild oats, yerba buena, red clover, horsetail, dandelion leaves or root, burdock root, alfalfa, kelp, red raspberry, or any other plant high in minerals
2 cups vinegar of your choice

Follow the steps for the basic herbal vinegar recipe.

## SUGGESTIONS FOR USE

Take ¼ to 1 tsp daily straight, mixed with water, or added to food. Combining vinegar with mineral-rich vegetables such as leafy greens makes the minerals in the vegetables more bioavailable. High-mineral vinegar is an excellent herbal ally to prevent loss of bone density and to support people with osteoporosis.

### Fuego

Fuego is based on a classic herbal folk remedy, also known as fire cider.* The basic ingredients are garlic, onion, ginger, horseradish root, and chili peppers. However, you may use your creativity and add other ingredients or omit others. Common additional ingredients include turmeric root, burdock root, astragalus root, thyme, rosemary, sage, and lemon or orange. If you don't have all the fresh ingredients, you may substitute with dried herb or powder. Because this is a folk medicine recipe, I normally don't measure the ingredients when I make my Fuego. I am giving an estimate of the amount of each ingredient, but feel free to adjust them.

---

* Fire cider is a folk remedy popularized by herbalist Rosemary Gladstar, which was adopted and used by herbalists across the world. In 2019, an herbal company tried to trademark the name Fire Cider and sued other herbalists for using the name. Fortunately, herbalists won the legal battle, and fire cider is no longer trademarked. To avoid legal repercussions, I called my fire cider "Fuego," but it's basically the same thing.

1 head garlic

1 large onion

1 medium-size horseradish root

1 medium-size ginger root

Cayenne or other variety of hot chili pepper (fresh or dried). Start with a small amount (one fresh chili or ½ tsp dried powder) and increase slowly to achieve the amount of heat you want.

Apple cider vinegar

Honey

1. Chop or grate the ingredients and add to your glass jar. You want the ingredients to be loosely packed and to fill up about three-quarters of the jar.
2. Cover ingredients with apple cider vinegar. Make sure the ingredients are completely immersed. If the lid is metal, insert plastic wrap between the jar and the lid to prevent rusting.
3. Label your jar with the ingredients and the date.
4. Option 1: Dig a deep hole in your yard. The hole needs to be deep enough to bury the jar completely. Place the jar in the hole and cover with dirt. Put a stone or some marker where you buried your jar, so that you can easily find it when it's done. After one moon cycle, dig it up and take it out of the earth.
5. Option 2: Store your jar in a place out of direct heat and light, and shake daily.
6. After one moon cycle (one month), strain out the plant material. Some folks compost the leftover vegetables and spices, which are called the "marc." I like to keep mine in a container in the freezer to add to soup stock. The marc should last a few months in the fridge, since they are soaked in vinegar. If you see signs of mold or spoilage, discard. Pour the vinegar back into a clean jar.
7. Add honey to taste to the vinegar. If you prefer a low-glycemic option, omit the honey.
8. Store in glass bottles. (Make sure you label your bottles!) It does not need to be refrigerated.

## SUGGESTIONS FOR USE

Fuego can be taken daily as a tonic. Suggested dose is ¼ to 1 tsp daily, or add it to food. For times when you are actively fighting an infection or are symptomatic, take ½ to 1 tsp every few hours.

## CONTRAINDICATIONS:

Do not take when undergoing surgery or if you are on blood thinners. It may irritate the mouth or mucous membranes. Avoid if experiencing gastritis or acid reflux. Do not take if you are sensitive to some of the ingredients, such as garlic or chili.

Entire books have been written about food as medicine.* I have learned much from my students about creative ways to incorporate herbs into food. Be creative and have fun!

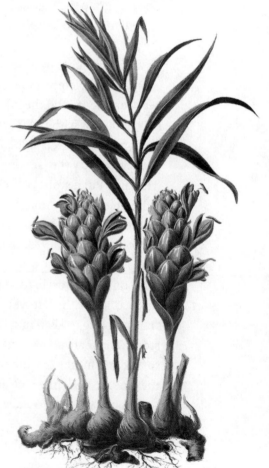

_____

* *The Herbal Kitchen* by Kami McBride is a great resource!

# Sandra M. Pacheco
## (she/her/ella)

> "Ancestral medicine is now inextricably part of my life and how I live rather than something I use when I am not feeling well. I now carry ancestral Indigenous practices all the time as protection, prevention, and spiritual practice."

Sandra (Mexicana, Chicana, and Indigena) was born in Los Angeles/Tongva territory and has lived in Northern California/Ohlone territory for more than half her life. Sandra has a doctorate in psychology, teaches extensively in the community, and leads workshops for therapists who serve predominantly Latinx and Indigena people. Sandra is a cofounder and steward of Curanderas sin Fronteras and deeply values that this medicine and knowledge be available and accessible to la gente. I first met Sandra when she became a student in the Curanderx Toolkit class, and we since have become friends, colleagues, and comadres on this path.

## SANDRA M. PACHECO SPEAKS:

My paternal grandmother, Doña Margarita Flores (aka Doña Mague), whom I am named after, was a healer. She carried ancestral medicine and practiced curanderismo. I witnessed her prepare herbs and foods for healing as well as offer limpias.

Curanderismo has always been part of my life, through my connection to Mother Earth, use of medicinal herbs, and food practices. As a young child I would blissfully spend time with plant relatives. But as soon as I started school, my time with plant relatives and my ability to hear them started to fade. Though I did not name my practice curanderismo at the time, I worked toward healing myself and family with herbs and food.

It was after a major soul loss that I returned more intentionally to ancestral medicine and recommitted my life to carrying on the tradition. I enrolled in the Curanderx Toolkit course, and this deeply launched me into reclaiming and recentering the practice.

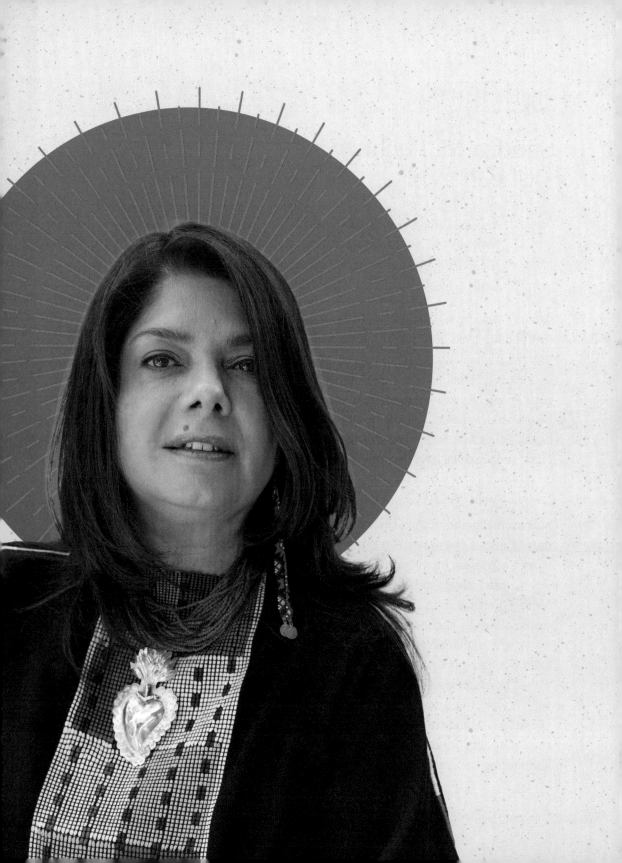

While I have been able to apply ancestral healing to my personal health and wellness through medicinal herbs and rituals as needed, the most important thing was to switch to living a life in relation to the ancestral medicine. It also has a political aspect to it. It is important as an activist to support our gente with affordable medicine, so we subvert capitalist models.

I have forever seared in my heart our first outing as Curanderas sin Fronteras at the Fruitvale Cinco de Mayo event. The line was endless, and we served over one hundred persons that day. We ran out of plants, and an elderly man came out of the line and went to get us more plants. The people we met knew the medicine, trusted the medicine, and knew how to engage with the medicine. Some knew what medicinal herbs they needed. One man cried as he shared it had been fifteen years since he had had a limpia. They wanted to know where we would be next. The need is great, and we are few.

It feels like the ancestral medicine was always there. However, now it is more amplified. Being able to offer limpias and education has been a tremendous blessing and honor. Seeing our gente desahogar [seeing our people experience cathartic release and unburden themselves emotionally] and have light enter their lives again is powerful. The opportunity to share curanderismo is a gift because it activates ancestral knowing in the next generations. A serendipitous blessing has been to see the younger generation in Oaxaca, who had begun to dismiss ancestral medicine, begin to return to their cultural healing practices. It has been an interesting dynamic where "extranjeros" of Mexican descent are returning to learn, which in turn has young folks in Oaxaca wondering what we are so interested in.

Curanderismo is not an easy path. For me, it is one that I am called to do and feel a tremendous responsibility to do so. The path is challenging and requires discipline, sacrifice, and an ongoing spiritual practice. I must protect my energy and stay healthy of mind, body, and spirit so I can be of service to others.

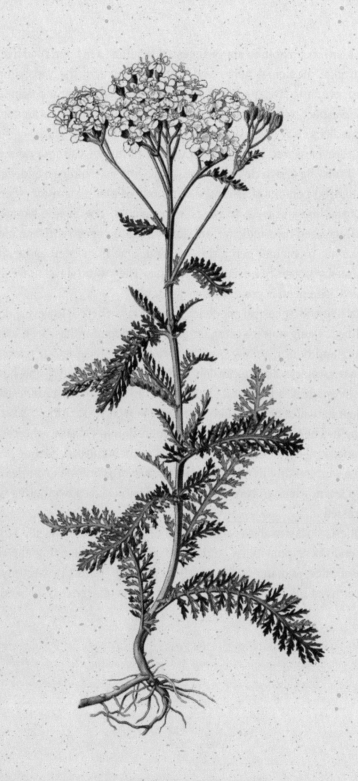

# CHAPTER 10

# Energy and Boundaries

Traditional cultural healing systems have different ways of describing the subtle, spiritual, and cosmic energies that influence human health. Hinduism describes the seven energy centers on the body called chakras. Traditional Chinese medicine is rooted in "Five Element" theory and maps out energetic pathways on the body called meridians. Ayurveda is based on a different theory of five elements and works with important energy points on the body called marma points. In modern holistic medicine, practitioners describe the body's aura or etheric field. Due to colonization, much of the knowledge of similar Anahuacan systems has been destroyed, stolen, and misinterpreted, or carefully hidden by keepers of the tradition. I have searched for and gathered parts of these teachings from my maestros, who each carry a different piece of this knowledge. These teachings have expanded my awareness of subtle energies in a system rooted in an Anahuacan cosmovision.*

The ancient Anahuacan people had very advanced astronomical knowledge. They carefully studied the movements of the sun, the moon, the planets, and the Pleiades. Their knowledge was recorded in the legendary Piedra del Sol/Sun Stone ("Aztec" calendar), whose true name is Huey Cuauhxicalli.** In the center of the Huey Cuauhxicalli is an image named Nahui Ollin, or "four movement." Nahui Ollin reflects the universal principle in which "four dynamic forces create the unique essence of every moment." This is a very sophisticated concept that describes the universal movement of energy into creation and form.[1]

---

* I am including a very brief introduction to the Huey Cuauhxicalli and Nahui Ollin here to connect the Anahuacan cosmovision to what I will share next about the four energetic bodies.

** *Huey Cuauhxicalli* translates to "Venerable Gourd of the Eagles," where the eagle (cuahtli) represents the sun. "Sun" represents the actual solar body, but also a "sun" is a cycle of 6,625 years.[2] In 2021, we experienced a major transition as one of these cycles ended and moved from the Fifth Sun to the Sixth Sun.

# Four Energetic Bodies

Nahui Ollin also expresses itself in the human experience, in which the dance of four energies creates a fifth entity. Human beings have four energetic bodies: the tonal, nahual, teyolía, and ihíyotl.* The interplay of these four subtle energy bodies gives birth to the fifth, our physical body, which is called the tonacayo. These four energetic bodies are in constant motion, creating continuous shifts within us. They are the subtle energies that create all that manifests in our physical form. For example, if one has an illness, such as a tumor, it first existed somewhere in one or more of the energy bodies. Historians have written about these energy bodies and how they relate to Anahuacan culture and cosmovision, yet rarely give instructions on how to apply this knowledge to our own health and well-being.[3] The first teachings I received on how to work with the four energy bodies came from Maestro Sergio Magaña Ocelocoyotl.

## Tonal

The word *tonal* is related to the Nahuatl word for the sun, *tonatiuh*. Tonal also corresponds to *tonalli*, which can be translated as "light of the day," but also refers to the energy of the day in the Mexica calendar on which a person was born. The energy of a person's birth date reveals their cosmic identity, or their gifts, abilities, and divine purpose. The tonal is our consciousness when we are awake and relates to our mind and our conscious thoughts.

The tonal is located around the head. It has a golden color like the sun and a warm energy. People who can observe subtle energies may see the tonal as a golden-yellow ring around the head, similar to a halo. When someone experiences trauma, shock, or strong emotions/aires, the tonal can be separated and lost from the body.[4]

Many rituals function to call the tonal back home to the body. The scent and power of aromatic plants help call the tonal back, which is why aromatic plants such as rosemary, rue, and pirul are always used in limpias. A way to observe a person's tonal is to look at the brightness in their eyes. The eyes of someone who has lost parts of their tonal through trauma, stress, and stuck emotions will

---

* In this tradition, the four energy bodies are not exclusively human but part of all beings, including animals, plants, rocks, and planets.

look dim or cloudy. Bright, clear, and alert eyes indicate the presence of a healthy tonal.

## Nahual

The word *nahual* translates to "who I really am."[5] Nahual also relates to *nahualli*, which means "what can be extended."[6] The nahual is our energetic body that governs our dreaming state. The nahual is ruled by the moon and the planet Venus. It has cooling energy and looks silvery like the halo around the moon.

During the day when we are awake, the nahual resides near our navel, and informs our gut instinct and intuition. However, the nahual does not remain static or permanently at the navel center. When we sleep, the nahual rules our dreaming state and switches places with our tonal and moves up to surround our head.

## Teyolía

*Teyolía* can be defined as "the energy around the heart," "divine fire," or "that which gives life to people."[7] As the spiritual energy of the heart, it is sometimes compared to the Christian concept of soul. Our teyolía bestows us human beings with feelings of love and other emotions and gives us the gifts of intelligence, personality, talents, and memory.[8] The teyolía supplies vital energy and is considered to be a precious resource that can be depleted under certain conditions. Many traditional practices exist to help preserve and protect the teyolía. When the teyolía is injured, it can cause mental instability and insanity.[9] Conditions such as sadness, depression, and melancholy are seen as imbalances of the teyolía. These conditions can be alleviated and the teyolía reinvigorated by using aromatic plants.[10] Our teyolía continues to exist after our physical body has died. After death, our teyolía may take different paths depending on the nature of our death. Most often, our teyolía will travel through Mictlan, the land of the dead, and eventually be reborn into a new physical form.[11]

## Ihíyotl

*Ihíyotl* can be translated from Nahuatl as "breath, respiration; life; sustenance."[12] This elusive yet powerful energy body dwells in the liver and is both gaseous and luminescent.[13] The ihíyotl is "the life force that comes from the subtle worlds and keeps matter alive,[14] and corresponds to passion, hatred, and other strong emotions.[15] One's ihíyotl attracts or repels other beings and may relate to what is called "animal magnetism."[16]

## MEDITATION:
## CONNECTING TO YOUR FOUR ENERGETIC BODIES

I created this meditation so that each of us can learn about our four energetic bodies through direct experience. Our energy bodies are intelligent and have much to teach us if we just take the time to listen and observe. As we gain more understanding of our energetic bodies, our healing work will have much more depth, as we are able to address the energetic cause of illness and disharmony.

To begin, create space for this sacred exploration. You may choose to light a candle and burn some medicine. Connect to your guides, ancestors, or inner curanderx. Set your intention to explore your energetic bodies and to learn more about them. You may choose to explore all four energetic bodies in the same exercise, or work with them one at a time.

Find a comfortable position sitting, standing, or lying down. Take thirteen deep breaths, breathing in through your nose and exhaling through your mouth. Allow yourself to shift into ensonación, a waking dream state.

## TONAL

Working with the tonal is best during daytime. To connect with your tonal, keep your eyes open. Attune to your waking-state consciousness, to your mind and thoughts. How would you describe it? What do you see or sense?* Feel your tonal as the energy around your head like a halo. You may choose to place your hands

---

* Tonal is related to but not limited to vision. For people who are blind or visually impaired, the tonal relates to their state of consciousness when awake, which may or may not involve sight.

on top of your head. What do you feel? Do you feel warmth or sense a particular color? Tune into your tonal. Does it have a message for you? What does it need from you?

When you feel complete, thank your tonal. Take four more deep breaths to transition out of the meditation or to the next energetic body meditation.

## TEYOLÍA

For this meditation, you may choose to keep your eyes open with a soft focus or close your eyes.

As you breathe, bring awareness to your heart center, the place where your teyolía lives. Feel into this area of your chest, your sternum, your lungs, and your heart. Breathe into your heart and sense the energy around your heart. You may choose to put your hands on your heart. Do you feel warmth or sense color?

Much energy is stored in our teyolía, including our emotions, memories, and connections to others. What emotions do you sense here? What memories may arise? In my teyolía, I can feel the connection to the people in my life whom I love. I can also feel the heavier energy of the relationships where there is conflict or hurt.

Our teyolía has lived many lifetimes and in many forms. As you sense into your teyolía, you may tap into ancestral memories or even past lives. Notice what arises.

The teyolía supplies us with our precious life-force energy. As you connect to your teyolía, observe the quality of its vitality. Does your teyolía feel bright and energetic or dull and listless? Or somewhere in between? Tune into your teyolía and ask whether it has any messages for you. Ask your teyolía what it needs from you.

When you feel complete, thank your teyolía and take four more deep breaths to transition out of the meditation or to the next energetic body meditation.

## NAHUAL

If you feel comfortable and safe doing so, close your eyes. Breathe into the area of your body right around your navel, your ombligo. You may choose to put your hands on your belly. Greet your nahual, your energetic body that governs dreamtime. We can connect to our nahual when we are awake but in a meditative or visionary state. What do you feel and sense in your nahual? Does it have a color or temperature?

The nahual often speaks in symbols, so notice what images arise in your mind's eye. Your nahual may take you on a dreamlike journey. Attune to your nahual and see whether it has any messages for you. Ask your nahual what it needs from you.

When you feel complete, thank your nahual and take four more deep breaths to transition out of the meditation or to the next energetic body meditation.

## IHÍYOTL

For this meditation, you may choose to keep your eyes open with a soft focus or close your eyes. The ihíyotl lives in the liver, which is located below the lower right rib cage. Breathe into your liver. You may choose to place one hand on your lower right ribs and one below it on your torso. Think about your life force, your passions, and your strong emotions. Notice the sensations and emotions that may arise. Do you feel temperature or notice a color? Does your ihíyotl have a message for you? What does it need from you?

When you feel complete, thank your ihíyotl. Take four more deep breaths to transition out of the meditation.

Take time to journal about what you experienced while attuning to your energy bodies.

# Las Trece Puertas/ The Thirteen Doorways

Another component of an energetic understanding of the human body is the teachings of las trece puertas, the thirteen doorways, which have been shared with me by Maestra Estela Román. Thirteen is a sacred number in curanderismo; and in Anahuacan cosmology, there are thirteen heavens. The number thirteen also relates to the movement of the sun, as every thirteen days (called a trecena), the sun rotates halfway on its axis to show a new face to the earth. Thirteen also relates to the moon, as each year contains thirteen moon cycles.

Our physical bodies also are connected to these cosmic patterns, and in our bodies we have thirteen primary joints or energy centers, which Maestra Estela calls doorways, or puertas. These puertas are places where energy moves into and out of the body. When we are in balance, our energies flow freely. When we are out of balance, energy can get stuck and cause problems, including pain, discomfort, or emotional distress. The thirteen primary puertas/joints are the occiput (base of skull) and the right and left ankles, knees, hips, wrists, elbows, and shoulders.

## EXERCISE: ATTUNING TO YOUR PUERTAS

This exercise is best done sitting or lying down. Create sacred space for this exploration and call on your ancestors and guides. Take thirteen deep breaths. Allow your body and mind to relax.

Take time to scan your body and focus your attention on your trece puertas/ thirteen doorways. Notice if your attention is drawn to a particular one. It may be where you feel pain, heat, cold, discomfort, or stagnation. What do you feel and notice here?

Gently move and stretch this puerta. Tune into this area and sense what emotions or memories you may be holding there. Breathe into this puerta and send it your love and healing energy. Attune to your puerta and ask whether it has any messages for you. When you feel complete, move slowly and take time to journal about what you experienced and any messages you received.

Both Doña Enriqueta and Maestra Estela have emphasized the importance of closing our puertas after they have been opened. Our puertas open when we have a limpia or a massage, or give birth. They can also open when we are experiencing stress, trauma, or strong emotions. In this exercise, our puertas opened as we brought our attention and focus to them. Therefore, to complete this exercise properly, we must close our puertas. A simple way to close each puerta is to gently squeeze each of your thirteen joints. If you can't comfortably reach any one joint, just imagine closing it. Close each of the trece puertas until you are complete.

# Understanding Our Boundaries

When we become aware of our subtle energy bodies and puertas, we can start to better understand our boundaries. Our boundaries relate to all the ways our physical and energetic bodies interface and interact with the rest of the world. Our universe is interconnected, so we are constantly swimming in the energy of the people and the world around us.

Boundaries protect our physical and emotional space from disturbance and harm. With strong boundaries, we try not to let anyone who may harm us into our personal space.* I may be walking down the street when a strange man starts to jeer at me and make inappropriate remarks. With a clear sense of my boundaries, I may cross the road to avoid him or turn around and walk away.

Our boundaries exist in our personal relationships as well. Maybe my coworker stands too close to me and puts their hand on my back. This gesture makes me feel uncomfortable. To honor my boundaries, I may take a step back or ask them not to touch me without asking permission. Our boundaries are also in motion. They can change from moment to moment depending on the environment we are in and the people we are around.

When my personal boundaries are in danger, I usually feel a tingling of fear in my stomach, which I feel is my nahual speaking to me. By activating a sensation in my gut, my nahual tells me that something is inappropriate or unsafe. It has taken years for me to learn to listen to my gut. I have been in many situations where I ignored the warning from my nahual, and I have suffered the consequences.

To set healthy boundaries, I have learned that I need to let go of being a nice girl. As a person who grew up Catholic, I have been deeply conditioned to be nice. Even though I am an adult woman in my fifties, I still struggle to change this deeply ingrained behavior. There is nothing wrong with being a nice person; in fact, the world needs more people who are kind and considerate. I am referring to the kind of "nice girl" behavior that always is trying to please other people. I was trained to be nice to people even when they are behaving inappropriately

---

* I deliberately used the verb "try" in the sentence "try not to let anyone who may harm us into our personal space." Sadly, we live in a world where people are attacked, violated, and even killed because they are Black, Indigenous, people of color, women, queer, trans, or of a different religion. I do not want to ever blame the victims of hate crimes for not having strong enough boundaries to stave off such an attack.

or making me uncomfortable. Many of us are conditioned to put other people's needs first and to ignore our own needs.

As I have learned to set my boundaries, I have needed to stop being a nice girl. It may be difficult to tell my coworker that I don't feel comfortable when they stand too close to me. They may respond with jest or anger. I am learning to live with the fact that people may not like me when I set my boundaries. Yet when I honor my own boundaries, I can avoid the detrimental effects of having my boundaries disrespected—headaches, digestive problems, insomnia, anxiety, and chronic illness. By honoring my boundaries, I also experience a sense of my personal power.

When I am around loved ones, my physical boundaries relax to allow them into my personal space. For those of us who are survivors of abuse or violence, our concept of healthy boundaries has often been distorted. A common tool for survival is to learn to tap into the energy field of the abuser, the addict, or the one who has done us harm. This behavior leads to codependence in which the boundaries between us and the other person are blurred, and we lose a sense of ourselves.

# Plant Allies for Boundaries and Protection

Many herbs are traditionally used for protection, and here I share a few of my favorites. As you work with these herbs, observe yourself and the way the plant interacts with you. What do you notice shifting in your body? How does the herb affect your energy level? Do you have more energy and feel less drained? How does working with your herbal ally change the way you feel when interacting with other people or going into public spaces? Do you feel less psychically sensitive? Are you able to tolerate situations that in the past would have thrown you off? Does it feel easier to speak up and use your words to defend your personal space?

# Milflor/Yarrow/Milenrama/Tlalquequetzal

*Achillea millefolium*

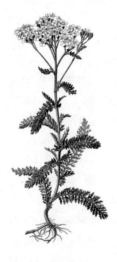

Yarrow is a plant native to Europe, Asia, Mexico, and the Americas. The Latin name for yarrow, *Achillea millefolium*, relates to the myth of the Greek warrior Achilles.[*] According to some versions of the myth, Achilles was dipped in a protective bath of yarrow as an infant, leaving only his heel vulnerable to attack.

The use of yarrow as a first-aid plant to treat wounds has been practiced for thousands of years by people across the globe. Yarrow is the first plant I use to stanch bleeding. With natural antimicrobial properties, yarrow also disinfects wounds. I use it topically to treat cuts, wounds, and punctures, and internally for conditions such as ulcers, hemorrhoids, and excessive menstrual bleeding.

Energetically, yarrow helps stop the bleeding of energy and promotes healthy boundaries. It protects us from unwanted energies and can also prevent our energy from bleeding into the space of others. I experience the medicine of yarrow as a shield of white light surrounding me. I have used it when in crowds or public spaces, from concerts to marches and protests. When I work with yarrow, I feel as though I am surrounded by a bubble of light, and I feel less affected by the energies around me.

I recommend yarrow as an all-purpose herb for boundaries. For those of us who tend to be psychic sponges, who too easily absorb the energies from people around us, I recommend using yarrow every day before going out into the world, or even before turning on your computer and reading the news or checking your emails.

Ways to work with yarrow include as tea, tincture, oil, liniment, flower essence, or amulet. Baths of yarrow are excellent for clearing out the energy of past relationships.

---

[*] Many of the scientific binomial names in the Linnaean system come from Greek or Roman cosmology. The names are often a by-product of colonization and heavily biased in western culture and thinking. I know this can feel alienating to people as many people's own ancestral worldview is not reflected in the scientific name. I recommend learning names for plants in the native languages of your ancestors.

# Tobaco/Tobacco/Iyetl/Piciyetl

*Nicotiana* spp

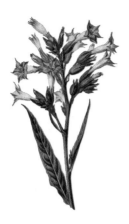

Since antiquity, tobacco has been used by Indigenous people on both sides of the US-Mexico border for ceremony, prayer, offerings, medicine, and doctoring. In ancient Mexico, images of tobacco flowers, gourds, and offerings are found in ancient rock art and in the codices.[17] Tobacco is one of the flowers decorating the famous statue of Xochipilli, the "prince of flowers." For parteras, tobacco is "a technology of birthing" and used to help facilitate labor and to call forth masculine energy to a newborn baby.[18] Tobacco has been traditionally used for many afflictions, including bites, burns, headaches, fatigue, and pain.[19]

Tobacco is a powerful guardian plant, which can be planted in your garden to help protect your home. In my experience growing tobacco, I have observed that tobacco knows where it needs to be to do its work. In my garden, for over fifteen years I had been cultivating a particular tobacco plant native to Mexico. Although I planted it in a certain area of my garden, every few years it chose to self-seed (plant itself) in other areas of my yard. One year, the tobacco self-seeded directly next to the main walkway into our housing compound. Any person entering our yard and home space had to walk right past the tobacco. The branches and leaves of the tobacco would literally brush against people as they entered our yard. I believe that this tobacco planted itself in that exact spot to help protect our household.

Tobacco can also be worn on the body for protection. I recommend making a small pouch of tobacco to put in your pocket or wear as an amulet. When I travel, I cut a fresh leaf of tobacco to put in my car. When I create altars for my herbal classes, I often include freshly cut tobacco leaves or even a small potted tobacco plant. The presence of tobacco helps protect both the people and the space.

Across the Americas, tobacco smoke is used for birth, healing, cleansing, and protection. When I am in need of a good cleansing, I roll cigarettes from my homegrown tobacco and blow the smoke on myself.* I often am guided to direct the smoke to certain places on my body where I feel stuck energy. Alternatively, if I haven't felt like smoking, I have burned the tobacco on a hot charcoal and blessed myself with the smoke.

Tobacco can be used as a flower essence for its protective and spiritual properties. It can also be infused into alcohol and used topically as a spray. It can be added to a limpia liniment. Because it has strong energy, I normally combine it with other plants.

Tobacco can be used safely topically by most people, but should be avoided or used with caution by pregnant people, children, and elders. Tobacco smoke can be irritating to people with respiratory challenges. Tobacco is a toxic plant, so never ingest it.

## Limpia Liniment

Herbal sprays or liniments are my favorite ways to work with plants for protection and cleansing. We can combine different plants in our liniments. I never measure the amount of plants in this recipe, so feel free to be creative and to work with what you have on hand and what is fresh and available. Plants that are aromatic, such as rose, lavender, rosemary, mint, cinnamon, or citrus, will give your limpia liniment a good scent.

### MATERIALS

- Fresh or dried herbs; options include ruda, romero, yarrow, rose, tobacco, mirto, mint, pericón, lavender, citrus, and cinnamon
- 16 or 32 oz glass jar with lid
- 80 proof (40%) alcohol (I prefer vodka because it doesn't have a strong scent, but you can use any hard alcohol, such as tequila, mezcal cane alcohol, or rum.)

---

* If you smoke homegrown tobacco, make sure you know whether the species you are growing is safe to smoke. Some species, including *Nicotiana rustica* (called "Aztec" or "Hopi" tobacco), are very strong and can have adverse effects.

## INSTRUCTIONS

1. Cut or chop up fresh herbs and pack them loosely in the glass jar.
2. Cover the herbs with alcohol. Make sure all herbs are submerged.
3. Cover and label your jar with the date and ingredients.
4. Shake the jar and put in your prayers and intentions.
5. Store the jar away from direct light or heat.
6. In one month, strain out the plant material. Give thanks to the plants and return them to the earth.
7. Add the liquid to a spray jar and label.

## SUGGESTIONS FOR USE

For daily protection, mist your body and your puertas. Spray indoor or outdoor areas to clear rooms or spaces. Incorporate it into self-limpias and meditation practices, and use it to enhance your work with the four energetic bodies. Do not take internally.

## SUGGESTED COMBINATIONS

- **Yarrow** and **rose** for emotional boundaries with loved ones
- **Yarrow** and **mugwort** for protection while dreaming
- **Yarrow, ruda**, and **tobacco** for a trinity of protective energy
- **Ruda** and **romero** for protection while traveling
- **Pericón, pirul, romero, mirto**, and **ruda** for working with all aires
- **Melissa, manzanilla**, and **rose** for calming and for working with grief

Enjoy the process of creating your own combinations and recipes. As you work with different plants, over time you'll discover which ones are most helpful for you.

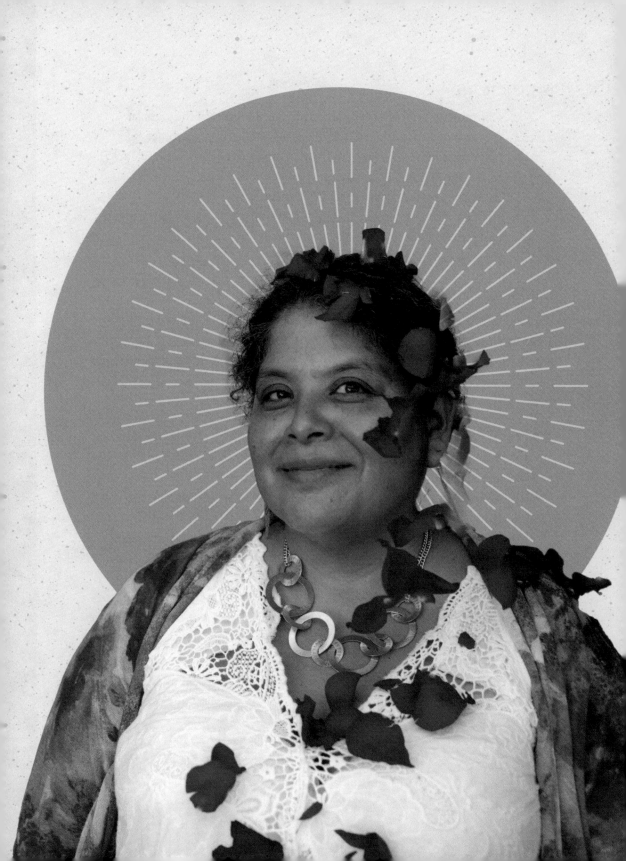

## SPOTLIGHT

# Brenda Salgado
## (she/her)

"If this is your calling, it is a tremendous joy to be of service in this way. Holding space and facilitating others finding their way, reclaiming lost part of themselves, and healing their ancestral line is so rewarding and contributes to this time of shift for future generations and our beloved Mother Earth. Also, remember that to be of highest service, we need to be constantly doing our own work, both as a modeling for others and so that we can walk this path with integrity, honesty, strength, and humility."

Brenda is Nicaraguan American of mixed European and Indigenous decent (Chorotega). Brenda was born and raised in Daly City/Ohlone territory, and both her parents come from small villages surrounding Volcan Masaya in Nicaragua. Brenda is grounded, compassionate, and wise and carries her medicine with humility and integrity. Brenda has been a regular guest teacher in the Curanderx Toolkit class, where she guides the Harmonizing and Healing with Roses ceremony. As part of her curanderx work, she offers limpias and energy and ancestral healings, and shares teachings about Indigenous prophecies.

### BRENDA SALGADO SPEAKS:

I knew as a young child that I was supposed to be a spiritual teacher and healer and said so to my mom. She assumed I wanted to be a nun, and I said no, it is more like a priest and also a healer.

In young adulthood, my beloved maternal grandmother, Maria, came to me in dreams and meditation. Abuela Maria shared that I come from a line of medicine women, and this was also my path. She said I needed to ask my mom and aunt for stories about her healing them and their siblings when they were children in Nicaragua. I learned that Abuela Maria healed my tía Carmen from a

serious illness which doctors said she would die from, and that she healed my uncle Chico of polio as a toddler. In both cases, she prepared herbal baths and wraps, and worked with various plant medicines.

My mother shared that my grandmother taught them to take medicinal herbal baths, she regularly prepared for them teas and purgatives, she used heat and cupping on sore muscles, and used an egg for cleansings. Some of the plants she used medicinally as well as in cooking included ruda, albahaca, epazote, romero, yerba buena, manzanilla, oregano, cilantro, canafistula. It has been a balm to my heart to learn that medicine was still carried so closely in the generations, and that it was my mother's generation where the break in this occurred. I had assumed it was lost farther back than this.

My exploration of this tradition initially was met by fear and misunderstanding from some family members. I also had an inadequate understanding about energetic boundaries and responsibility, so I took on other people's energies and was even healing others out of my own life force, becoming ill as a result. I needed to establish healthy reciprocity in order to honor myself and my gifts as I offer service in my community.

I advise those starting down this path to make the time to slow down and listen from time to time. Listen to ancestors, to the precious plantitas, to Mother Earth, to Creator, to your own higher self. There are so many nonhuman relations and guides who wish to support us. Cultivate and trust in your own intuition and sovereignty, and honor that in others as well. Be wary of those who say they know what is best for you, push you to do something when you are not ready or choosing this willingly, or wish you to cede your sovereignty and inner knowing to them.

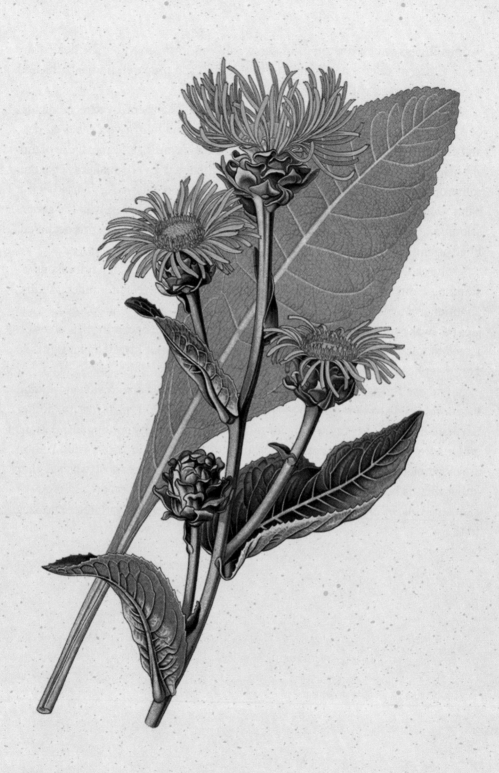

## CHAPTER 11

# Dancing with los Aires

We have to face the aires, which are really teachers. For myself, I went through many layers of working with the fear, with anger, and each time it's like peeling an onion to go deeper and deeper. Working with each layer creates more consciousness and also much change in our lives. When the energy that was lost in that dynamic, that aire, is released, it makes room for our own energy of light to come back. When we do that, we start to blossom and bring our gifts to the world.

—Marcela Sabin

The healing philosophy of curanderismo evolved from a close observation of nature. Our abuelas y abuelos carefully studied the natural world around them. They understood that human beings were not separate from the natural world but instead were an intrinsic part of it. They knew that their physical and emotional bodies were always influenced by nature and the cycles of the cosmos. They knew that they, as human beings, also had a responsibility to tend to nature to help maintain balance and harmony.

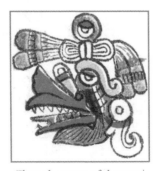

Ehecatl, energy of the wind

# Introducing los Trece Aires

According to teachings developed and shared by Maestra Estela Román, there are trece aires—thirteen winds.[1] They relate to the trece puertas/thirteen doorways on our physical body. Every one of us dances with each of the thirteen aires at some point in our lifetime.* When los aires are present, we can feel the energy we label as "emotions." Los aires come on suddenly like a whirlwind, or they may have been hanging around with us for years. Los aires can affect our minds, and we may feel confused or disoriented, have a hard time focusing, or be plagued with racing thoughts. Los aires may present as air-like sensations in the body, such as gas, bloating, and burping. Pain that moves around the body is also a sign of wind. Los aires can cause many different symptoms in the physical body, including (but not limited to) headaches, cramps, muscle tension, nausea, or insomnia. Aires can accumulate in the abdomen, which can lead to chronic health problems. Most of us recognize the aires we carry. Often we become so accustomed to the presence of los aires in our lives that we start to claim ownership of them. We may say things like "my anger" or "my fear" or "my sadness."

The concept of los aires, or "the airs" or "the winds," is part of a complex ancestral cosmovision. The ancestors of this tradition studied carefully how energy moved on earth, in the cosmos, and in our bodies. They knew that our bodies were a microcosm of the universe. Los aires are energies that exist in the cosmos and also can exist in us. Trudy Robles says, "Los aires are not organic to us," which means that they are not part of our essential nature but outside forces that move through us. When aires move through us, they can cause disequilibrium that can manifest physically, such as by our catching a cold or feeling pain.** Unlike emotions as understood in a westernized view, aires are not just a psychological concept but real energetic entities that Maestra Estela calls "cosmic

---

* To study los aires is to study a mystery of the universe. I am a humble student of los aires on this lifelong path of study. I am sharing my understanding of los aires, which is based on the teachings of Maestra Estela Román and shared here with her permission. My thoughts on los aires are also informed by my own exploration of los aires in myself and my conversations with other curanderx. My particular viewpoint is just one way to approach a study of los aires, and each curanderx has their own understanding and contributions to this body of knowledge. Maestra Estela continues to develop her teachings, and I recommend her book *Nuestra Medicina* for people who want to learn more.

** "Mal aire" is a common diagnosis. There are many ways to catch mal aire, such as being exposed to a draft or to cold wind.

winds."* According to her teachings, the struggles we face in life are related to the aires. No matter how hard we try, we can't make the winds disappear; they are simply a part of life here on Tonantzin.[2]

Los aires relate to the element of air, and, like Ehecatl the wind, los aires are normally in motion. It is their nature to move around us and through us. When los aires are in balance, they flow gently, but when they are out of balance, they may blow so powerfully that they knock us over. Sometimes the winds freeze. We feel stuck, unable to make changes or move forward in our lives. Other times los aires take up residence inside us, invite their friends, and have a party. We feel swallowed by a torrent of emotions inside us. When los aires are not in balance, they can block our happiness, creativity, and life force. We may feel heavy, numb, depressed, or sick. We all carry our own individual aires as well as the aires of our ancestors.

Los aires can also act like children who trick us and play games with us. They lurk in corners waiting to trip us when we're not vigilant. We may think we have evolved because we have "done our work" and are no longer susceptible to their influences. Then suddenly life happens—we lose our job, our partner leaves us, or we have a falling out with our best friend. In all kinds of situations like this, los aires spring out of their hiding places, chase us around, and laugh in our face with triumphant glee. They snicker at us: "Ha, ha, you thought you were so mature and grown up! I'll show you!" We're once again consumed by any one of them—such as jealousy, anger, fear, or anxiety.

Like the wind, los aires can move quickly from one person to another. Los aires can dance between family members, friends, and coworkers, and they can swirl through communities. Have you ever noticed that when you are around someone who is really mad, you may also start to feel agitated and angry? Once I spent time supporting a friend who was going through an anguishing heartbreak. After sitting and listening to her for about an hour, I suddenly burst into tears when I got home. I had not been feeling sad, yet I felt as though I had been touched by her aire of pena. When strong aires blow, they can impact the entire collective. A great example of this was at the beginning of the COVID-19

---

* Some aires are elemental guardians of nature, which Maestra Estela calls "aires de la tierra." These aires guard sacred spaces such as springs or mountains. Traditional people maintain a respectful relationship with these aires by performing certain rituals and offerings. When we don't respect the guardians of nature, they can cause problems for us. Unfortunately, many of us have forgotten how to tend to them.

pandemic, when people all around the world starting hoarding toilet paper. Within days, all toilet paper quickly disappeared from grocery store shelves. As los aires of susto and miedo were activated by the shocking reality of a global pandemic, people the world over felt this fear and began to panic. In fact, by studying the human response to the entire COVID-19 pandemic, we can all learn much about the way aires blow through the collective. When working with my own aires, I always take time to ask myself, "Is this aire coming from me, from the people around me, or is it in the greater collective?" The good thing is that no matter where the aire originated from, we work with it the same way in curanderismo.

Many of the practices we have in curanderismo, such as limpias and baños, are to help us work with and release our aires. To do so, we must call on the energy of Huitzlampa and tap into the energy of our inner warrior. Working with our aires takes much effort, strength, courage, and endurance. Sometimes the aires are stubborn and don't want to go. They dig their claws into us and refuse to budge. Other times we are attached to our aires and have a hard time releasing them. We may have based our entire identity on our aires—for example, thinking "I am an angry person" or "It is my nature to be worried." Releasing our aires is hard work. When we release our aires, they can make us burp, fart, cry, shake, scream, vomit, or feel paralyzed. The aires are no joke! But when we can finally let them go, we feel lighter, happier, healthier, more energized, and more creative. We have managed to free ourselves from their invisible prison, and all of our precious life force that it took to handle them is now liberated. We have also freed los aires, so that they may return to the dance of the cosmos.

One way to learn about los aires is to study the nature of Ehecatl, the wind. The cosmic winds possess all the same qualities as wind does in nature. Sit outside and observe the movement of air in your environment. How does the energy of wind move? What effect does wind have on the environment? What does a strong wind feel like? What does a cold wind feel like? What does lack of air movement feel like? Los aires also move in the air in our homes, such as air conditioning, drafts, or forced heat.

One of the most important ways to learn about los aires is by studying ourselves. When an aire is present in our lives, we can welcome it as our teacher and invite ourselves to be curious about its nature. Here are some questions that I have found helpful to ask myself each time one or more of los aires is present in my life:

- What does the aire feel like? Where do I feel the energy of this aire in my body? How would I describe the physical sensations?
- How would I describe the degree and force of movement of this aire? Is it like a gentle breeze or a strong wind? Does it feel frozen, stuck, and stagnant?
- Does this aire feel hot or cold? Or a mixture of both? Where on my body do I feel the heat or cold?
- How does this aire affect my thoughts? Are my thoughts racing or looping? Do I feel spacey? Am I checked out?
- How does this aire affect my energy level? Do I feel tired or wired? How much of my precious life force is taken up by managing this aire?
- What is this aire teaching me about myself? When have I experienced this aire before? Is this an aire present in my family and ancestors?
- What do I need to do to work with and release this aire?
- How do my energy and mood shift when I am able to release this aire? What else may have changed in my life?

Duality is a fundamental principle in our ancestral cosmovision. The universe is full of examples of duality: day/night, heat/cold, young/old, waking/sleeping, sun/moon, and fire/water. Los aires also are a part of this duality. When we are struggling with an aire, we can say that the energy is out of balance, or existing in an unloved state.* When an aire is out of balance or unloved, it can cause us to suffer; yet when the same aire is balanced and loved, it can be our teacher and a gift.

---

\* Thank you to Trudy Robles and Carmen Hernandez, who collaborated with me to create a handout on los aires. They conceptualized the idea of duality as it relates to los aires as well as contributed information about which area of the body is affected by each aire.

# Caution: Aires Crossing!

Los aires are not just psychological concepts but living, intelligent forces in the universe. Los aires seem to be particularly attracted to spaces where they are being studied or discussed. I have noticed this phenomenon in the classroom whenever we hold the class on los aires. Just speaking the names of los aires out loud seems to call them into the classroom. Everyone in the room will start to feel unsettled as the cosmic winds blow through the space. As the aires dance around us, they may abruptly grab any one of us and insist that we tango with them. Students have reported that all of a sudden they feel incredibly sad or fearful or full of anguish or taken over by whichever aire is present.

I am not sharing this to scare you but to prepare you for what you might experience as you read about los aires. In this moment as I am writing, I can feel los aires swirling around me. The aires that showed up today directed me to include these words of caution. As I write about each one of los trece aires, I myself am dancing with each one and recalling times in my life when they were present. I am needing to work with a lot of medicine and take breaks to get through writing this chapter.

Remember, los aires aren't malicious or harmful. They are our teachers, our friends, and gifts from the universe. My advice is to start by grounding yourself. Light a candle, say a prayer, and make an offering to the cosmic winds. Burn medicine. Move slowly through this section at the pace that is just right for you. Take time to reflect and digest not just what you are reading but what is activated within you when you read about los aires.

# Fear and the Stress Response

Curanderismo has evolved as practice of resilience and resistance through a history of genocide and colonization. Curanderx have become experts at treating people who suffer from violence and trauma. When someone is faced with a threat of danger or violence, a normal human response is to feel fear. The ancestors of this tradition observed the nuances of fear and identified three aires that relate to it: susto, espanto, and miedo.

Human beings, like all other animals, have a hardwired physiological response to a threat of danger. Whenever our brain faces a real or perceived threat, it responds instantaneously by activating the sympathetic nervous system. The sympathetic nervous system mobilizes energy and responds to the threat by activating a fight, flight, or freeze response. The stress hormones cortisol and adrenaline are secreted, which activate a cascade of physiological effects in the body. The heart rate increases, blood pressure rises, and breathing is accelerated. People feel more alert, and their senses are sharpened. Blood flow increases to the heart, brain, and muscles, and glucose is released into the bloodstream. This all provides extra energy and strength to navigate the threat, to fight or to run away ("flight"). Sometimes when faced with a threat, we might freeze up, become immobilized, or even play dead (as is the case with possums). In the freeze response, we feel numb and checked out, and we disassociate or energetically separate from our bodies and from the present moment.

This fight-flight-freeze response to stress is invaluable when we face real danger. Our bodies give us the energy and focus to survive life-threatening situations. These are the situations where people can accomplish superhuman things, such as escaping from a burning building or lifting a heavy automobile to rescue one's trapped child. However, the same physiological response is activated by everyday stressors that are not life threatening. We may be stuck in traffic and notice that our muscles are clenched and our blood pressure is rising. Our brain does not distinguish between fleeing a natural disaster and stressing about a work deadline. The stress response is also activated by worry, anxiety, and negative self-talk. Any of the thirteen aires can activate the body's stress response, and especially those aires that relate to fear. When we experience chronic susto, miedo, or espanto, our nervous system endures a continual state of stress and arousal. Chronic stress can exhaust and deplete the body and contributes to many common illnesses such as hypertension, diabetes, autoimmune disorders, and cancer.

# Plant Allies for Working with los Aires

Some of the most profound and personally helpful knowledge that I have received on this path of healing is that of los trece aires. As someone who walks with deep ancestral, generational, and personal pain, it has been so helpful for me to relate to painful emotions as messenger energies and teachers, to continuously be in an awareness of how I feel, and to be in the ongoing practice of helping emotions move. I also work closely with my ancestors who guide my life. I tend to their altar and talk with them throughout the day. They help me do my work to face difficult situations and transmute stagnant emotional pain (aires) so that pain is not left here with me, on earth, and/or passed to others.

—Batul True Heart\*

Fortunately, Tonantzin generously provides us with countless herbs and flowers that can support us when we are stressed, fearful, or facing any of our aires. Every single plant has the potential to help us. Elder Mexican curandera Doña Chucha, who specialized in treating susto and espanto, taught that any plant, even a simple piece of grass, could help us balance our aires. All plants are a gift from Tonantzin; we simply need to pray to the plant and ask it to help us. All of the traditional ways of working with herbs in curanderismo, such as in limpias, baños, and the temescal, are excellent methods of addressing los aires.

In herbal medicine, certain categories of herbs excel at supporting our body's response to stress, and therefore are also helpful when working with los aires. One category is herbal nervines, which nourish and tonify the nervous system. Nervines can help relax and release tension and stress from the body, and calm anxious and worried thoughts. Nervines help us recover from any aire that arouses the nervous system and stimulates the fight-or-flight response. Examples of nervines are manzanilla, wild oat, and melissa.

Another category of herbs called adaptogens support our strength and resilience when we are facing stress. Adaptogens help the body adjust to multiple stressors and mitigate the stress response so that it has less of a detrimental

---

\* Batul True Heart has designed a remarkable flower essence line that has a remedy to address each aire. See https://maasomedicina.bigcartel.com/.

impact on the body. Adaptogens work by supporting different physiological systems of the body, including the nervous, immune, and endocrine systems. Adaptogens are highly regarded plants found in cultures all around the world. Well-known adaptogens include ginseng, tulsi, ashwagandha, reishi mushroom, and rhodiola.

Strong emotions, especially anger, relate energetically to the liver/ihíyotl. Many herbs that are tonic to the liver help us release anger and other strong aires that may be stored there. When working with herbal nervines, adaptogens, or liver tonics, we can take them as teas, tinctures, vinegars, or cordials, or use them in food.

Flower essences are also excellent allies that can support our work with all of los aires. Flower essences activate the harmonizing duality of each aire. For example, if we are working with the aire of miedo/fear, we take a flower essence that increases courage, the harmonizing duality of fear. Flower essences are taken in drop doses internally; used in misters, baths, or liniments; or applied directly to the skin.

# Los Trece Aires

> We, the curanderos, don't just give people tea or an herb. We look for the origin of the problem, whether it's pain, sickness, grief, loneliness, fear, timidity, anger.[3]
>
> —Doña Enriqueta Contreras

## Susto/Fear/Shock

Susto is caused by the experience of a sudden shock. There are different degrees of susto, ranging from minor to major. For example, if someone is crossing the street and a car runs a red light and almost hits them, this person may experience a mild susto. They may feel shaky, scared, and disoriented. Yet with the right care (such as calling a friend for support, having a good cry, taking a bath, or drinking a relaxing tea), the person may find that their susto resolves in a few hours or few days. If this same person is hit by the car, they will have suffered a major susto. Major sustos take longer to heal. Some major sustos take years or even decades of regular treatment to resolve. Posttraumatic stress disorder is the psychological term for chronic susto. For example, survivors of war, violence, oppression, or abuse can suffer from chronic susto.

Energetically, susto can be both hot and cold. In the moment of a traumatic event, susto can generate heat (sweating, racing heart, increased circulation, and so on). Over time, a susto can become frozen in the body, and the heat of the original susto is encapsulated by cold. Symptoms of susto include loss of appetite, sudden weight gain or loss, sleeping problems, exhaustion, anxiety, depression, difficulty focusing, feelings of disassociation, pain or tension in the body, or digestive problems. People who suffer from susto will often say that they "feel off" or "don't feel like themselves." When we experience a susto, the shock forces part of our tonal to leave our physical body. The treatment for susto always involves calling the tonal back into the body.

In her workshop on susto y espanto, Doña Chucha shared that in the past, her community held an elaborate and effective ceremony to cure a person who was suffering from severe susto. This all-night ceremony required twelve people to pray together, light candles, and administer tea to the sick person. The group would then move in procession to the place where the susto occurred (such as the site of an accident). Together the community would help release the sombra, or shadow, of the sick person.

Hearing this story from Doña Chucha taught me that healing severe trauma is possible with the participation of many hands and hearts, not just of one solo curanderx. What could this kind of ceremony look like in our world today? What if we gave the gift of our time and energy collectively to help our community members heal?

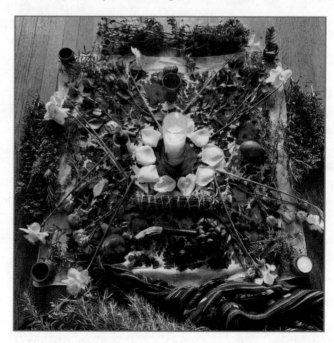

## HERBAL ALLIES

To treat susto, we can work with herbal nervines and adaptogens. We work with herbs that help us feel safe, grounded, calm, and stable, which are expressions of the loved state of susto. We also use herbs and practices to call the spirit back into the body.

- **Wild oat** is a nourishing nervine that restores our nervous system when we've been exhausted by chronic susto and stress.
- **Reishi mushroom** is an adaptogen that is calming, grounding, and deeply nourishing. It helps stabilize the body, mind, and spirit after trauma. It also increases the body's resilience to stress.
- **Cempohualxochitl** soothes the emotions and calls the spirit back into the body.

# Espanto/Supernatural Fear

Espanto is a type of fear that comes from encountering supernatural forces such as ghosts or spirits of nature. Animals and children are especially prone to espanto. When we experience espanto, our nahual senses energies that may not be visible in the physical plane,* and we may feel spooked and unsettled. Espanto tends to feel cold.

I learned of another interpretation of espanto from Doña Chucha. She described it as caused by impressions we see over time, such as being repeatedly abused. According to her, espanto can be like a shadow that hangs over a person and can manifest in flashbacks. During a flashback, people relive a past experience of trauma. People experiencing flashbacks can completely lose touch with the present moment and may be overtaken by images and sensations that aren't present physically but feel real.

---

* Although some people have the ability to see spirits. Also, sometimes supernatural activity is so strong that things occur on the physical plane, such as books falling suddenly off shelves or items mysteriously disappearing.

## HERBAL ALLIES

Because espanto is often about being oversensitive and vulnerable to outside influences, we work with herbs that promote healthy boundaries. We use herbs that help us feel safe and protected, which is the loved state of espanto. For flashbacks related to espanto, I often use herbs that treat trauma and herbs that bring people back into their bodies and into the present moment.

- **Yarrow** strengthens boundaries and will help protect from unwanted energies.
- **Ruda** protects against visible and invisible entities.

# Miedo/Fear

Miedo relates to common fears most of us face as humans, such as fear of illness, death, and the unknown, as well as phobias. Miedo is sometimes but not always caused by a susto. For example, if someone is attacked by a dog, they may suffer a susto from the attack that leads to a long-term fear (miedo) of dogs. By contrast, someone may suffer from arachnophobia (fear of spiders) even though they have never experienced a susto related to spiders. Nightmares may also be related to miedo. Like susto, miedo can present as a combination of heat and cold.

## HERBAL ALLIES

To harmonize miedo, we want to work with plants that increase courage, confidence, and serenity, which are qualities of miedo's loved state.

- **Manzanilla** is soothing and comforting. Its sweet and gentle energy has an affinity for children and animals. It can be used in a dream pillow to quell nightmares.
- **Mirto** has been traditionally used to treat susto, miedo, and nightmares.

# Coraje/Anger

Anger is a natural response to many life circumstances. Anger can arise when we feel threatened, when our boundaries are crossed, or when we face unfairness, abuse, discrimination, or injustice. Like fear, anger has a physiological response in the body that can propel us into a fight-or-flight response. Our body releases adrenalin, which tightens muscles, increases heart rate, and raises blood pressure. Anger is often described as hot, as in "hotheaded" or "hot-tempered."

The aire of anger can be like a tornado, destroying everything in its path. When overtaken by the wind of coraje, we can lose control of ourselves and potentially harm ourselves or others. However, when we try to control and repress coraje, it can fester inside us, leading to both physical and emotional health issues. The liver is the organ that relates to the aire of anger, and it can be injured by either excess or repressed anger. When we take herbs that stimulate the liver, they can potentially activate our hidden and buried anger. As the buried anger comes to the surface, it may even express itself physically as a rash or other symptom of heat.

When we learn how to dance with the aire of anger, it can be a powerful ally. Anger is a source of raw, untamed energy that can be channeled into positive change and used as a source of action and creativity. When in its loved state, coraje can express itself as passion, motivation, and determination. Coraje can teach us how to let go, lighten up, and cultivate acceptance and gratitude.

## HERBAL ALLIES

All herbs that support the liver (called bitters or hepatics) can help treat coraje. Herbal nervines can cool a hot and agitated nervous system.

- **Dandelion** root is a gentle liver tonic. It is grounding and nourishing and can be helpful for calming angry agitated states. *Diente de leon* translates as "teeth of the lion" and can encourage us to roar when we have been repressing our anger.
- **Scullcap** soothes our nerves and calms us down when we are quick to anger.

# Resentimiento/Resentment

The aire of resentment is a close relative of the aire of anger. Whereas anger can be hot and inflammatory, resentment is cool or smoldering. When anger is not expressed, it can transform into resentment or bitterness. Bitterness and resentment often arise when we feel that we have been mistreated or treated unfairly. I have noticed that I feel resentful when people take up too much space or act from a place of entitlement and privilege. Usually, the aire of resentment arises in me when I am unable to speak up. When the aire of resentment blows, we may feel disempowered and victimized.

Resentment is cold, although often there is heat buried beneath its surface, like a hot ember encased in ice. Resentment can lead to stagnation of movement, which can manifest physically as problems in the joints (puertas), such as arthritis and pain. When we experience resentimiento's loved state, we step into our power, speak our truth, and take responsibility for our lives.

## HERBAL ALLIES

To work with this aire, we can use herbs that help unblock stagnant emotions, help release bitterness, and cultivate forgiveness and understanding. Because resentment is related to anger, all herbs that work on the liver can also be used.

- **Estafiate** works on the liver and helps us release stored anger and resentment.
- **Willow** helps us let go of bitterness and feeling like a victim. It helps us forgive and empowers us to take responsibility for our own lives.

# Celos/Jealousy

Jealousy is a complex, tricky aire that seems to prefer the company of other aires. When the aire of jealousy shows up, it likes to invite its friends fear, anger, resentment, and sadness. We often think of jealousy as relating to intimate relationships, but jealousy can be present in all kinds of relationships.

As an aire, jealousy can be hot, strong, and overpowering. When the wind of jealousy is with us, it can cause obsessive thinking and irrational behavior.

In certain cases, jealousy can lead to increasing suspicion, controlling behavior, and even violence. When expressed in its loved state, celos can look like self-confidence and self-love. Celos teaches us how to cultivate an open heart and to practice nonattachment.

## HERBAL ALLIES

To work with this aire, we use herbs that increase self-love and self-esteem, as well as those that connect us to a divine source of unconditional love.

- **Burdock root** is sweet, grounding, and nurturing, and helps build our vitality and sense of self. It clears negativity, including strong negative emotions. Burdock also works on the liver and can soften the anger that often accompanies jealousy.
- **Rose** is the quintessential plant of love! Roses have the highest vibration of any plant. When we work with rose, we are infused with the high vibration of love, which can dissolve the aire of jealousy.

# Envidia/Envy

Envidia is closely related to celos. When the aire of envy blows through us, our attention is pulled outside ourselves. We do not feel satisfied with ourselves, and we desire the qualities or possessions of other people.

Envidia can teach us to love and accept ourselves. Envy can inspire us to follow our dreams and create the kind of life we want to live. When envidia is sparked by competition and scarcity, we call forth the qualities of its loved state, which are appreciation and graciousness. Envidia can teach us to be generous, to share what we have with others, and also to collaborate and work together.

## HERBAL ALLIES

To work with this aire, we use herbs that soften strong emotions and open our hearts to receiving and giving love.

- **Holly** flower essence helps neutralize strong negative emotions directed toward others, such as envy, by connecting to a source of universal unconditional love.

- **Tulsi** or **holy basil** is an Ayurvedic herb that connects us to the divine feminine force. It fills us with so much love that aires such as envidia just melt away. As an adaptogen, it gives us strength, nourishment, and mental clarity.

## Egoismo/Egotism

The aire of egotism is one that is sometimes hard to recognize in ourselves. Our ego likes to drive our behavior but stay hidden from view in the unconscious mind. Egotism is self-centered, self-absorbed, and beyond fault. Egoismo relates to an inflated sense of self-importance, and the culture of white supremacy and patriarchy thrives on it. Racism and sexism (and all other isms) are both individual and collective aires of egotism.

Egotism also relates to low self-esteem. Low self-esteem can be the result of a dominant culture that tells us we aren't good enough. For people who have experienced systemic oppression, fostering a positive sense of self is a revolutionary act.

Egoismo has a different temperature quality depending on the way it is presenting in a person. A person with an overinflated ego may be loud and domineering, and take up too much space, which are characteristics of heat. A person with low self-esteem may be quiet, passive, and timid, which are cooler energetic qualities. Depending on the other aires present, the degree of hot or cold may vary, or both may be present in the person. The loved state of egoismo is healthy self-esteem, humility, and balanced leadership.

### HERBAL ALLIES

To work with egoismo, we use herbs that cultivate a healthy, balanced ego.

- **Sunflower** flower essence helps build self-esteem and self-confidence. It helps us take up the right amount of space in our personal ecosystem. It can also be used to help people who take up too much space.
- **Tobacco** flower essence helps us understand our place in the sacred web of life. Tobacco essence can boost low self-esteem by revealing our divine self and purpose. Tobacco can also help soften an over-

inflated ego by helping us understand our interconnectedness and interrelationship with all living beings.

# Verguenza/Shame

When I think about verguenza, I wonder how present this aire was in our ancestral cultures that were not dominated by oppressive forces. Today, the aire of shame is a powerful tool of colonization, patriarchy, white supremacy, and organized religion. These systems condition us to believe that we are unworthy, despicable, or sinful. If who we are, how we act, or whom we love falls outside the rigid social norms, these systems will unleash the aire of shame on us.

Although the aire of shame may be activated by forces outside us, it can be very insidious. It is easy to internalize this aire and allow it to take us over. When we are consumed by the aire of shame, we feel as though something is inherently wrong with us. We feel inadequate and worthless, and can be swallowed with low self-esteem and self-deprecating thoughts.

The loved state of verguenza is unconditional self-love and self-acceptance. For me, regular self-care nurtures my sense of self-love. As I tend to my emotional wounds and scars, I foster compassion and acceptance for these parts of myself.

## HERBAL ALLIES

To work with verguenza, we use herbs that help heal underlying trauma that causes shame and also herbs that cultivate self-love and acceptance.

- **Melissa** brings sweetness and has an affinity for healing sexual trauma and shame around sexuality.
- **Rose** has high vibrations that call forth the energy of love, including self-love.
- **Buttercup** flower essence helps us recognize our inner and outer beauty and encourages self-love.

# Culpa/Guilt

Guilt is the twin aire of shame. They are often inseparable and enjoy swirling around together. Whereas the aire of shame makes us believe there is something inherently wrong with us, its sibling, guilt, arises when we feel that we have done something to cause harm or hurt. Shame says, "I am a bad person"; guilt says, "I did something wrong." Guilt can be a normal part of our moral compass, helping us take responsibility for our actions and how they impact others. If we lie or steal, feeling remorse can be a healthy response. When the aire of guilt blows, it can inspire us to take corrective action. We can apologize, make amends, and change our behavior.

However, the aire of culpa can sometimes blow too strongly and throw us off balance. We may feel guilty for our emotions even when they are justified. We may feel guilty for our thoughts, our actions, or our desires. Like shame, the aire of guilt can be activated by forces outside ourselves. In my life, the Catholic Church activated strong winds of both guilt and shame in my life, particularly around sexuality. When I was a young woman at Catholic school, the teachers and nuns drilled into me that sex was sinful unless it happened in the context of heterosexual marriage. As my own sexuality blossomed, I felt ashamed of my sexual inclinations, and I felt guilty for expressing them. I internalized both of these aires deeply, and they still blow around me from time to time.

## HERBAL ALLIES

To address the aire of culpa, we work with herbs that support self-forgiveness and lighten up self-judgment.

- **Mint** is a great energetic cleanser, which can help release any of the aires, including culpa. It is brightening and refreshing and helps us lighten up. Mint helps bring mental clarity and a fresh perspective to situations where we feel stuck.
- **Pine** flower essence helps people who feel overly guilty and beat themselves up. Pine helps us stop being so hard on ourselves and to feel our perfect, divine nature.
- **Milk thistle** helps us forgive ourselves. It releases the barbs we direct at ourselves, such as guilt and self-blame.

# Pena/Sorrow

Pena is a cold aire that relates to a state of grief and arises when we experience loss of all kinds. Loss and grief are both inevitable parts of the human experience, yet many of us have lost touch with our ancestral rituals that mark death and loss.

Grief is a sacred process that takes time and patience. We are often not given, or do not give ourselves, the time and space to fully grieve. When we do not fully grieve, the energy of the aire of pena will manifest in other ways, often presenting as health issues. Grief relates to the lungs, and unresolved grief will often manifest in respiratory problems, such as asthma or bronchitis.

Loss and heartbreak are invisible wounds. If someone breaks their leg, their leg cast will signal to the world (and to that person) that they are injured and in the process of recovery. But we can't see heartbreak in others, so we may not comprehend that people are grieving. When we dance with pena, we may feel depressed, anxious, or exhausted; have a hard time sleeping; or experience pain or other symptoms in the body. In its loved state, pena helps us accept our loss, grieve, let go, and move on.

## HERBAL ALLIES

There is no magic pill or herb that can take away the pain of heartbreak and grief. While we grieve, our herbal allies can be part of our support system. They can soothe, comfort, and hold us through the process.

- **Cempohualxochitl** is like a ray of sunlight on a dark, cloudy day. Its bright orange and yellow blossoms comfort us during times of grief.
- **Magnolia** or **yolloxochitl** ("heart flower") has been used in Mexico for centuries as a remedy for a broken heart.
- **Bleeding heart** flower essence helps ease the pain of a broken heart. It encourages the flow of emotions so that our hearts can heal.

# Tristeza/Sadness

The aire of tristeza is a kind of sadness that can relate to what we call melancholy or depression. When tristeza blows around us, we feel cold and lonely. Unlike the aire of pena, tristeza is not always activated by a loss. However, unresolved pena can lead to tristeza. When tristeza is present, we may feel flat, apathetic, and as though we have lost our enthusiasm for life. We may feel disconnected from what brings us joy. In its loved state, tristeza is happiness, contentment, and enthusiasm for life.

## HERBAL ALLIES

To address tristeza, we work with herbs that help us lighten up and cultivate playfulness and joy, as well as herbs that help us feel loved and supported.

- **The Grandmother Plant** (*Tagetes lemmonii*) brings the support of an abuela who is loving yet firm. When we are feeling sad and lonely, it can help us connect to our female ancestors as a source of guidance and support. It connects us to our wise inner elder.
- **Bougainvillea** flower essence brings peace, ease, and playfulness. It helps us shift our perspective and expectations and cultivate an attitude of gratitude.
- **Borage** flower essence brings hope and optimism. Borage lifts our spirits when we feel heavyhearted.

# Angustia/Anguish/Anxiety

The aire of angustia is a compelling dance partner who loves to sweep us off our feet. From a physiological perspective, anxiety relates to the nervous system's sympathetic stress response of fight or flight. With anxiety, the stress response is always turned on. Whereas stress is triggered by a real immediate threat, anxiety often does not have a clearly identifiable trigger.

In its loved state, angustia feels like love, peace, stability, and trust. To work with the aire of angustia, we use herbs that call in these harmonizing qualities. In addition to working with herbal remedies, many other self-care practices can help alleviate anxiety, including exercise, meditation, breath work, massage, baños, self-limpias, acupuncture, and psychotherapy.

## HERBAL ALLIES

Most people working with the aire of angustia would benefit from both herbal nervines and adaptogens, which calm the nervous system, quiet the mind, and build strength and resilience. We can also work with herbs that support energetic cleansing and protection.

- **Nettles** nourish the entire body and also restore exhausted adrenal glands. According to herbalist Karen Rose, nettles can heal the blood lineage, which makes them a useful ally for working with anxiety that we inherit from our parents, grandparents, and ancestors.
- **Pirul** is a strong energetic cleanser and can help release all aires, including angustia.
- **Pericón** offers protection, relieves anxiety, and helps us connect to inner and outer resources for healing.

# Gracias a los Aires

Dancing with los aires is part of the cosmic dance of life. Gracias a los aires who continue to teach me about myself, about nature, and about the world around me. They have taught me the importance of la medicina and how to work with the elements of nature to rebalance myself time and time again. I give thanks to the herbal allies who steadfastly support me each time I am blown around and thrown off balance by los aires. I offer a deep bow of gratitude to Maestra Estela Román for her years of dedication to the study and teaching of los aires. Her teachings have deeply enriched my life and the lives of countless others of her clients and students.

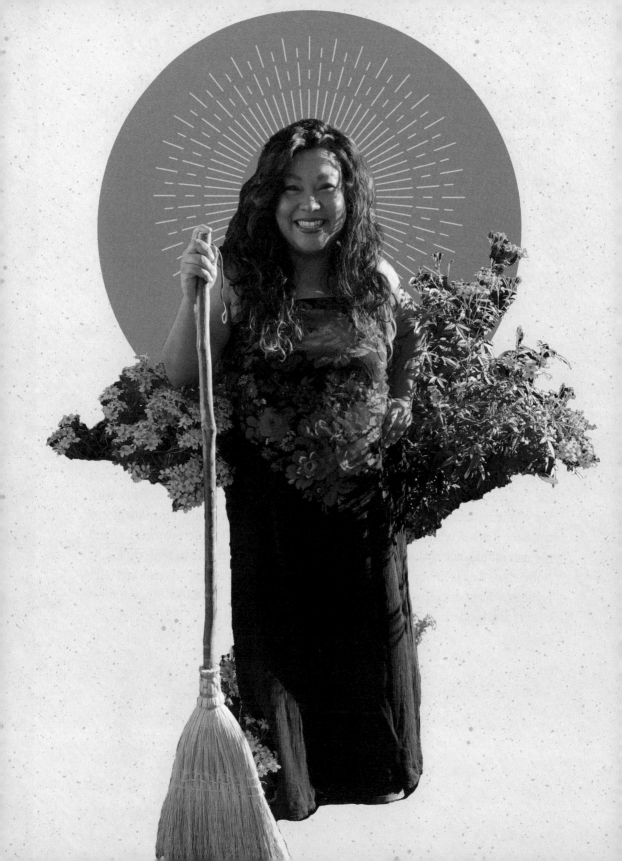

# SPOTLIGHT

# Angela Raquel Aguilar
## (they/she/we)

> "We are all our own curanderxs. This healing path is messy, painful, nauseating, beautiful, transformative. It is a lifelong commitment, and it truly is chosen for us. Follow the signs, follow your gut, follow your heart, and follow the plants."

With ancestral roots in Mexico and New Mexico, Angela was raised by a single mother and grandmother in Southern California/Kizh and Tongva territory before moving to Huchiun/the East Bay as a young adult. Angela is a mother, community health worker, scholar, and full-spectrum traditional birthkeeper. They focus on issues of sexual, reproductive, and healing justice in their educational and organizing work and are the cofounder of Nueva Luz (re)Birth and Family Care, which offers education and consulting to birthing people framed in a decolonized and re-Indigenized approach to birthwork. Angela applies their ancestral medicine practices to support parents and birthing people in preparing for conception, pregnancy, birth, and parenting. They help people get ready for the birthing ceremony through integrating and teaching the lessons of the limpia ceremonia. They also support survivors of childhood sexual abuse on the journey of healing through birthing.

I met Angela in 2012 at an event called Earth Skills: Restoring Health, Childbirth, and Independence from Industrialized Medicine. This gathering was a convergence of like-minded people, many who shared a passion for remembering and reclaiming our ancestral medicine. After I met Angela, she signed up for almost every class at my school, and over the years we have become friends. I admire the passion they bring to their personal healing work and the way they transform their own trauma into medicine that they can share with others.

## ANGELA RAQUEL AGUILAR SPEAKS:

I was raised by my grandmother until I was twelve years old. She learned yerbería from her mother. My abuelita is also an energy worker (divination and medium). She taught me the basics growing up: how to relate to plants and plant medicine, how to work with energy and dreams, and how to use intuition. She also taught me about food as medicine and is a brilliant kitchen alchemist.

I came to curanderismo as part of my healing journey. I had gotten lost (or rather, had taken an underworld detour) after my abuelita left, experienced a range of sexual assaults and trauma from childhood to young adulthood, and used drugs and alcohol as a way to heal. When I decided to intentionally begin a healing journey at age twenty-six, I sought my ancestral ways, my abuelita's teachings, to bring me back home. I relearned curanderismo as I healed my trauma. Around the same time, I became a birth doula. I began to see the overlapping teachings in birthwork and curanderismo, in particular the work of a limpiadora de aires.

By walking with my ancestral medicine, I have learned to trust myself, a huge blessing as a survivor of childhood sexual abuse and assault. Trust is what is taken from us survivors. Moving through the path of curanderismo has helped me navigate out of places like depression and anxiety . . . I still experience those aires, but I don't live in them for months and years like I used to in my youth and young adulthood. I have learned to love life.

My advice for people on this path would be to stay organized and work with others. Form a healing circle or a healing collective, or whatever formation suits your folks. Teach each other, support each other, practice on each other, grieve with each other, and work it out with each other. Healing together comes first. Curanderismo is not a professional orientation—it is a way of life.

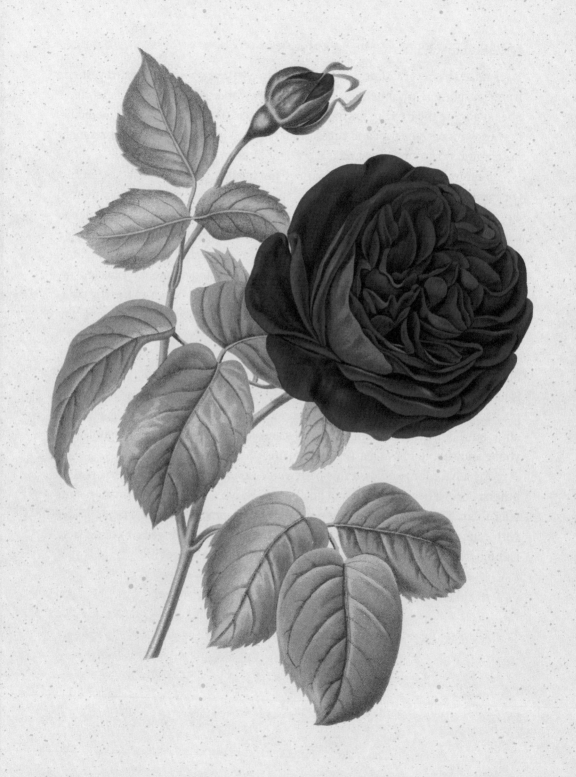

# CHAPTER 12

# Cleansing Ourselves: Limpias and Baños

We clean our cars, we clean our houses, yet we have forgotten how to clean our spirits.[1]

—Laurencio López Núñez

Traditional cultures all around the world have practices for cleansing of the body, mind, and spirit. Yet many of us living in a colonized world have lost touch with these practices and have forgotten how to take care of ourselves this way. We move through the world accumulating energies from the people and world around us. We breathe in polluted air. We eat food full of chemicals and pesticides. We read about tragedies in the news. We experience prejudice, discrimination, and injustice based on our gender, our gender identity, the color of our skin, whom we love, or how we pray. We survive a natural disaster, but keep living with its effects. We fight with our loved ones. We experience loss, heartbreak, and suffering of all kinds. Yet many of us haven't learned to take the time to care for our sacred body and spirit by cleansing ourselves of these energies.

The limpia is a traditional Indigenous practice of cleansing and healing. Patrisia Gonzales describes limpias as "a ceremonial and energetic framework for restoring wellness based on Indigenous ways of knowing and experiencing the cosmos within and nearby our bodies."[2] In Mexico, the practice of the limpia pre-dates European contact and has endured in spite of more than five hundred years of colonization. The limpia has been and continues to be a powerful tool for addressing the trauma of colonization and all subsequent prejudice, discrimination, and violence caused by colonialism. Like many other aspects of Mexican traditional medicine, over centuries the knowledge was protected and preserved in people's homes and families.[3]

The limpia is an opportunity for cleansing, restoration, and renewal. In the limpia, we can let go of the aires we have been harboring. We can cry and scream and release our anger, fear, resentment, shame, or sadness. The limpia helps us release harmful or toxic energies we may have picked up from food, air, people, or the collective. We can release our past traumas and even traumas we inherited from our ancestors. The limpia is not only about letting go of what we no longer need but also about calling in fresh energies. Limpias can renew our sense of vitality and creativity.

Limpias are also helpful in honoring the transitions we go through in life, such as birthdays, starting or ending a relationship, or changing careers. Receiving a limpia gives us a chance to both acknowledge and ritualize these major transitions. Each major transition in our lives is both a death and a birth. For example, if someone is graduating from college, the phase of their life as a student is coming to an end. Yet at the same time, this graduate may be moving and starting a new career, which is a birth of a new phase of their life. Transitions can be challenging when we have a hard time letting go of the old or when we cannot yet see or sense what is coming next. Rituals to honor our transitions will help the process go more smoothly and gracefully.

Another very important function of the limpia is to call a person's lost energy back into their body. According to my maestras, every time we suffer a susto or strong aire, part of the energy body called the tonal can leave our body. Without our tonal fully present, we can suffer from soul sickness or soul loss. All the elements of the limpia—the scents, the sounds, the songs, the touch, and the prayers—help call the lost tonal back into the body. During the limpia, we use our voice to invite our soul back home to our body. We call our name out loud and say, "Regresa! Regresa a tu casa!" "Come back! Come back to your home [your body]!" We welcome home the lost parts of ourselves into a space that is safe and sacred. When our lost soul finds its way back home, we feel reenergized, inspired, creative, and happy. The light of our renewed tonal shines through our eyes. Our eyes look clear, and our faces seem to glow.

Every curanderx will have a different style of doing a limpia and different tools that they use. No two limpias are ever the same. The limpia is a very creative and dynamic process in which the curanderx connects to their divine source and follows the stream of energy as it flows. Sometimes the energy flows gently; sometimes it is forceful. I have learned to always expect the unexpected in a limpia. I have seen people cry, scream, vomit, and experience temporary paralysis as part of the process of release.

When we receive a limpia from a curanderx, it may last anywhere from a few minutes to a few hours. The length of time depends on the way the curanderx works and how deep they take us into the process. Once at a health fair, I received a limpia that lasted about five minutes. I stood in the July heat under the shade of a large cottonwood tree while the curanderx recited prayers and blessed me with the smoke from their popoxcomitl. As she moved the popoxcomitl across my body, from head to toe, from front to back, a cloud of copal smoke engulfed me. I closed my eyes and listened to the sound of the rattle and the rhythmic chanting of their prayers. It felt good to receive this blessing. I left feeling a little lighter, but did not experience a major shift. Other limpias can be much more intense and last for hours.

Learning how to give limpias to others is beyond the scope of this chapter or this book. I think the best way to learn is through mentorship with another curanderx. There is no substitute for hands-on experience and direct guidance from one's teacher. The aires and other energies that may be released can be overpowering, and people who are not well trained can risk hurting themselves or the people they are working with.

Doña Enriqueta once shared a story about a foreign woman who was visiting her. This woman claimed to have a lot of experience working as a healer and asked to assist Doña Enriqueta during one of her limpias. Doña Enriqueta didn't think the woman was prepared to help with the limpia, but the woman insisted on accompanying her. They were working with a client who was an archeologist and had been working at Monte Alban, a sacred archeological site, when he fell ill. Doña Enriqueta suspected that he was afflicted with an aire de la tierra, a spirit that was likely the guardian of Monte Alban. During the limpia, strong aires started to release from the client, who started to moan and shake. Doña Enriqueta turned around to ask the foreign woman for help and noticed that she was passed out flat on her back. The aires that were releasing from the man were so powerful that they had knocked her out. Doña Enriqueta told us that she then needed to take care of both her client and the woman. For me, this story is a good warning about how we must be well trained and well prepared before giving limpias to others.

# Self-Limpias

An important part of my curanderx toolkit has been learning how to give myself a limpia. Energetically cleaning ourselves and tending to our aires should become part of our regular practice. We cannot wait until we see a curanderx to take care of ourselves. If we aren't doing our regular maintenance work with ourselves, we create much more work for the curanderx. They then need to deal with all our garbage that has been accumulating for months or years, which I think is an unfair burden to place on our healers.

For maintenance, we can do a self-limpia once every moon cycle. Any time of the month is good, or we can align with the phase of the moon to amplify our intention. The dark moon helps us to release, the new moon is a good time for planting the seeds of a new cycle, and the full moon intensifies the energy of what we are trying to accomplish. Sometimes when we are under more stress or are dealing with many of our aires, we might need to do a limpia every week or even every day. I often do not plan my self-limpias in advance, but tend to myself when I start feeling funky or out of balance, when I need to let go of something, or when I need to clean myself off energetically.

In her workshop on susto and espanto, Doña Chucha recommended that when we experience any kind of mal aire, even if it is minor, we must tend to it right away. This could include receiving upsetting news, getting into an argument, or being rejected for the job we applied for. As soon as we can after experiencing the aire, she advised finding the nearest leaf or branch and giving ourselves a quick limpia. I have found that to give myself a quick limpia, if I am outside around plants, I don't even need to pick the plant. Sometimes I just rub my hands or even my head through its leaves and branches. Sometimes I just hug a tree. Other times I lay on the ground and release the aire back to Tonantzin.

Trained curanderx offer limpias to support people in all kinds of situations. I have given people limpias for birthdays, graduation, and other important milestones, such as starting a new job or becoming a parent. Limpias can help with the process of grieving the death of a loved one or for recovering from illness or surgery. There are a few situations in which I would not recommend a limpia, such as when someone is seriously ill or emotionally fragile. Sometimes in these situations a limpia can be helpful, but at other times it can be too physically depleting or emotionally draining. In these circumstances, I have instead offered blessings, restorative practices, and prayers for healing.

# Limpia Tools

Whether we are receiving a limpia from a curanderx or doing our own self-limpia, many of the elements are the same. Although many curanderx work with the same basic tools, such as fresh herbs, an egg, and copal, each curanderx will at the same time incorporate their own unique medicina in their limpias. I will share some of the most common elements that are part of limpias in curanderismo.

## Egg/Huevo

In limpias, a whole raw egg is rubbed over the body to absorb unwanted energies. The egg is a universal symbol representing fertility, regeneration, and new life; when rubbed on the body, it acts like a psychic vacuum cleaner. As we move the egg over the body, we can listen to the sound of the egg, which can give us clues to where energy is stuck. Some curanderx use the egg as a diagnostic tool. After using the egg for a limpia, they crack the egg into a clear glass of water. They read the bubbles and filaments of the egg white and pay attention to the shape and color of the yolk. For example, if there is a dark spot in the yolk, this could be a sign of an illness in the physical body. I have heard stories about the egg absorbing so much energy that it became cooked like a hard-boiled egg. If they are available, eggs from free-range chickens work best.

As the egg absorbs much heavy energy, it is important to dispose of it properly after the limpia. I have been taught to bury the egg in the earth or to flush the contents of the cracked egg down the toilet.

One night after the limpia session in the Curanderx Toolkit class, I decided to bring all the used eggs of my students home with me so that I could bury them in my yard. There wasn't a good patch of earth near the classroom to bury the eggs, so I thought bringing them home would be the best way to dispose of them. When I arrived at my house with the bag of used eggs in my hand, I opened the gate to our backyard. Right on the other side of the gate was a skunk. We were both startled to encounter one another, and the skunk did what it does when it feels threatened. It sprayed me and the bag of eggs I was carrying. I immediately dropped the bag of eggs to the ground and stripped off the outer layer of my clothing before running upstairs to my apartment. That evening, I spent hours trying to clean off the skunky smell.

This encounter with the skunk taught me an important lesson: be careful not to take responsibility for other people's energetic waste. (Or, more bluntly, let people deal with the disposal of their own shit.) I had willingly carried fifteen eggs home, full of multitudes of aires and funky energy. The skunk told me, "Danger! Don't bring that into your house!" After the incident with the skunk, I no longer carried other people's used eggs home with me. When I work with a client, I normally ask them to take the egg home and bury it in their yard. This gives them the opportunity to complete the final step of their limpia, which is to offer the energies back to Tonantzin. If my clients can't bury their own egg, I will crack the egg, flush its contents down the toilet, and compost the eggshell.

## Lemon

As an alternative to the egg, some curanderx use a fresh lemon. The use of the lemon was introduced to me by Doña Doris Ortiz Ortega and Doña Felipa Sanchez. They taught that the lemon can be used similarly to the egg and is rubbed over a person's body to draw out aires and unwanted energies. The bright, cheerful scent of the lemon is uplifting and can relieve both sadness and depression, so by working with a lemon, we bring its healing qualities to the limpia. The most useful thing I learned about the lemon was that it can be reused three times! To recharge the lemon between limpias, simply drop the lemon on the floor. Lemons are often in abundance in Huchiun/the Bay Area, as many people in California have lemon trees, so it is often easy to find a fresh lemon. I recommend experimenting with the egg and the lemon to see which one works best for you.

## Broom Made of Fresh Herbs and Flowers

Along with the egg or lemon, another very common element of most limpias is a bundle of freshly cut herbs and flowers. Fresh, aromatic herbs have been used since antiquity in Mexico for cleansing, healing, and ceremony. Each plant reflected a part of the cosmos and was associated with certain sacred energies, such as pericón corresponding to Tlaloc.[4] Aromatic plants were used to repel unwanted entities from the water and the underworlds, to help cure ailments of the teyolía, and to help bring back a lost tonal to the body.[5] Flowers were especially sacred and considered to be a representation of the cosmos.

When I gather the herbs for my self-limpia, I begin by making an offering to the plants and asking their permission to harvest some of their leaves and branches. I say my prayers and ask the plants to support my healing intentions. I often sing a little song to the plants when I am harvesting them. As I harvest, I am doing a gentle pruning, which is like giving the plants a haircut. Many of the plants that we use, such as rosemary or the Grandmother Plant, benefit from regular pruning, as it can encourage new growth. When harvesting, I make sure to gather only a little bit from each plant so that I leave plenty for the birds, insects, and pollinators.

Once we gather our fresh herbs, they are bundled together to make a small broom either tied with string or simply held tightly in the hand. Herbs that are aromatic and high in essential oils, such as basil, rosemary, rue, or pirul, are often used for limpias. Depending on the plant, its scent can be calming or invigorating. Other scents bring a sense of happiness and peace. The vibrant aroma of all plants helps call our spirit back into our body. As we rub fresh herbs on our bodies, we absorb the essential oils through our skin. They can help stimulate circulation and move stagnant aires and energy. Fresh herbs, when rubbed across the body, are excellent at cleaning our energetic body.

Rosemary, basil, mirto, pirul, lavender, feverfew, rue, and pericón are all commonly used, although it is best to work with what is locally available. The

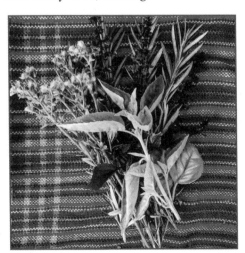

general rule is that the herbs must be fresh. Once I taught the Curanderx Toolkit in Minnesota in the late winter. As a person from the Bay Area, I was used to the luxury of having many good medicinal plants growing year-round. When I arrived in Minnesota, none of the plants I was accustomed to gathering from my garden for limpias were available. I knew we would have to find a creative solution. I spoke with my host and asked what aromatic plants were available, and she immediately answered, "cedar." We drove out to the countryside and harvested bundles of cedar to use in our limpias. They worked perfectly, and everyone enjoyed being cleansed with the cedar trees, which were an integral part of their natural environment.

Fresh flowers are also often used for limpias. I have been taught to add a few flowers to each bundle of herbs I make. Each flower brings color and its own healing properties to the limpia bundle.

## Sahumador/Popoxcomitl

The popoxcomitl (which translates to "smoking pot" or "incense burner") is a sacred tool that has been used in Mexico since ancient times. The popoxcomitl, also called the sahumador or copalero, is the vessel for burning copal or other plants to create smoke. According to Maestra Chicueyi Coatl, "The Sahumador is the means through which we communicate with our Ancestors, the Cosmos, and everything far and near."[6] The smoke is also used for protection, cleansing, and blessing, and to harmonize the energies in people and in environments. Doña Velia from Teopotzlan, Mexico, teaches that the popoxcomitl represents the womb and that the copal smoke is the umbilical cord that connects us to the cosmos.[7]

Some curanderx have strict protocols for the ways to work with the popoxcomitl. Similar protocols are taught as part of Danza traditions to sahumadorx whose sacred responsibility is to care for the popoxcomitl. I respect all these traditions and the ancestral wisdom behind them. Trudy Robles taught me and other sahumadorx how to use ocote (resinous branches of pine trees) to light the sacred fire in the popoxcomitl. Other curanderx use fast-lighting charcoal to ignite the fire. I think the most important thing is to treat the popoxcomitl with respect. When working with the sahumador, we are carrying the sacred fire. It takes time and practice to learn how to be in good relationship with the fire element. If we are not careful, we can accidentally burn ourselves or others. In the limpia, we use the popoxcomitl along with copal or other herbs to offer our prayers to the sacred energies and to keep the space clean energetically.

# Copal

Copal is the resin from the tree genus *Bursera* and has been used since antiquity in Mexico as a ceremonial and medicinal plant. The *Bursera* genus includes other trees sacred to other cultures, including frankincense and Palo Santo. The word *copal* is derived from the Nahuatl word *copalquahuitl*, which translates to "incense tree." The smoke of copal has been used traditionally in many kinds of ceremonies to communicate with the cosmos and to send messages to the ancestors. Copal has a high vibration; it brings positive energies to the space and helps lift our consciousness.[8] There are different types and colors of copal, which have different meanings and purposes. Although copal has been harvested sustainably for generations in Mexico, the copal tree is currently endangered and at risk. Please obtain from ethically harvested sources.

# Floral/Herbal Water

Another way to keep the limpia space energetically clean is to use floral or herbal waters, which I call limpia liniments. (See chapter 10 for a limpia liniment recipe.) Working with a water-based herbal spray is sometimes a good alternative to working with smoke. Sometimes we can't use fire or create smoke because it is prohibited in the spaces where we are working (such as hospitals or schools). Sometimes people have respiratory conditions such as asthma or chemical sensitivities that make them sensitive to smoke. In California during wildfire season, I have found that most people don't want to be exposed to more smoke, even in rituals.

Normally, I like to use both copal smoke and a limpia liniment, as they have different healing qualities. When we work with water for cleansing, it can feel cooling and invigorating, whereas to me smoke feels warmer and more sedating. I like to use the limpia liniment in a spray bottle, so I can freely mist the space and the people in the space. For people who are sensitive to smells, water by itself is a great way to cleanse. I like to dunk my bundle of herbs in a fresh bowl of water and sprinkle it around the space or on myself.

# Musical Instruments

Drumming, music, dance, and song have always been an integral part of ceremonies and celebrations in Mexico. Many curanderx incorporate sound and music into their limpias and other healing rituals, such as the temescal. During a limpia, a chorus of sounds—the drum's heartbeat, the spirited sonaja, and the pure, heartfelt song of the curanderx—weave together to transport us to a space that is sacred, magical, and healing.

Modern research on music therapy has proven it to have numerous benefits for physical and emotional health. Music decreases anxiety, depression, pain, and blood pressure. Studies on people going through chemotherapy and radiation found music to decrease nausea and vomiting and lower overall distress and anxiety.[9] Drumming has been shown to decrease inflammation, boost the immune system, and benefit people with posttraumatic stress disorder and dementia.[10]

In Nahuatl, the word for drum is *huehuetl*, which means an ancestor or an elder, and its beat resonates in our bones, where our ancestral memories are stored. The drum connects us to our own heartbeat, to our ancestors, and to the heartbeat of Tonantzin. The deep resonance of the drum can help us feel grounded and stabilized. At the same time, the strength of a drumbeat can be energizing and can break up stagnation in our physical and energetic bodies. A steady drumbeat can help shift us into a different state of consciousness, signified by an increase in alpha brain waves. Alpha brain waves signify a state of peace and relaxation and are also present in the brains of people who meditate.[11] Achieving an altered state of consciousness is important in the limpia. To be fully present for our healing, we need to shift out of our everyday mindset where we are planning, making lists, worrying about the future, or ruminating about the past. In my experience, hearing the drum transports me into a sacred place where I have acute awareness of the present moment. When we reach this state of being present and relaxed, true healing can take place.

In my self-limpias, I like to drum at the beginning when I pray and invite in the energies of Nauhcampa. I sometimes hold the drum close to my body so I can feel its vibrations. A fierce drumbeat can help me tap into buried emotions. Often the tempo of my drumming will speed up as I am releasing, and a fast, strong drumbeat often accompanies me when I cry, wail, and scream. The drumbeat slows down as I reach completion of my release and move into a state of rest.

In limpias, we can also use rattles for prayer and for song. The vibration of the rattle helps move stagnant energies. Similar to that of a drum, the sound of the rattle can help shift our state of consciousness. A traditional rattle made from the seeds of the ayayotl tree (*Thevitia peruviana*), called ayoyotes, is often used by both curanderx and danzantes. When in movement, the ayoyote seeds sound like rain or like the timbre of a rattlesnake.

## Song

The human voice expressed through song has healing and transformative power. Songs tell stories, awaken memories, lift our spirits, and soothe our hearts. Songs can catalyze action and unite people in struggle, grief, prayer, and celebration. The song of the curanderx is a sonic prayer. The curanderx sings to our weary spirit, to our broken heart, and to each organ and cell of our sacred body. They sing a lullaby to our tenderhearted inner child. Their loving voice can touch our spirit and open the flow of emotions. Their song can hold us while our heart cracks open, and their voice is a balm to soothe our wounds and our broken heart. The song of a curanderx can call a lost soul back home to the body.

I encourage everyone who is practicing self-limpias to sing! It can be very liberating to sing out loud. Allow the sound to flow from your heart. Express the feelings deep inside you that are hard to put into words. Sing to los aires, to your body, to your ancestors, and to Tonantzin. This is your healing song, and it is not meant to be judged or criticized. We can also make a soundtrack for our self-limpias. What songs help you connect to your grief, your anger, your joy?

## Chocolate/Cacahuatl/Xocolatl

Indigenous people in Mexico have been cultivating chocolate for thousands of years. It is considered a sacred plant, which was gifted to the Nahua people by Quetzalcoatl. Chocolate has many ceremonial and medicinal uses. When we have received a limpia, we may feel vulnerable after engaging in such deep healing work. Maestra Estela teaches that eating a little bit of chocolate brings warmth and helps us transition back into the world. Chocolate, mixed with herbs such as pericón, cinnamon, vanilla, or rose, can also be taken as a warm beverage.

## Herbal Tea

After we complete our self-limpia, it is important to stay warm and preserve our body's heat. At this time, we should avoid cold drinks and cold food. A good option is to drink a cup of hot chocolate or herbal tea. Any herbal tea can work; here are a few suggestions:

- Cinnamon + rose (warming and heart healing)
- Ginger + burdock root (warming and grounding)
- Yerba buena + lavender (invigorating; improves mental clarity)
- Manzanilla + melissa + pericón (calming and soothing)

These are all some of the most common tools used in limpias and self-limpias. Other tools that are used include stones, feathers, scissors, obsidian tools, and other musical instruments.

# Self-Limpia Process

A self-limpia can be simple or elaborate, depending on your time and intention. There is no right or wrong way to do a limpia. It is a dynamic and creative process, and each of us will develop our own unique way of working. Listen to your inner curanderx and the guidance of your ancestors. Follow the flow of energy as you begin to dance with your aires. The energy may rise and fall in waves, with moments of intensity and moments of rest. Listen to your body and trust yourself to know when the process is complete.

Here are some possible steps based on how I most often work with both myself and my clients:

1. Set your intention. Take some time to journal about your intention before you begin.
2. Create sacred space.
3. Find a space that is private and safe. It is best to do your self-limpia in a space where you won't be interrupted.
4. Gather the tools you will be using: the egg, lemon, herbs, sacred smoke, drum, rattle, and so on.

5. Pray and welcome in the energies of Nauhcampa, Tonantzin, and your ancestors and spirit guides. Greet and acknowledge the ancestors and living Indigenous stewards of the land you are on.

6. Take some time to breathe and ground yourself. Scan your physical body/tonacayo and notice where you feel pain, discomfort, blockages, or aires. Check in with your four energetic bodies. Pay particular attention to the state of your tonal and teyolía. Does your tonal feel bright or cloudy? Do you feel heavy emotions in your heart/teyolía? Choose which tool or tools you are drawn to work with.

7. To work with the egg or lemon, rub it directly on your body. Start at the crown of your head and then move down your body. Rub firmly, as if you were scrubbing a pot. A raw egg can surprisingly withstand an amazing amount of pressure. Give attention to each of your thirteen puertas/joints and to any other place on your body that needs it. Breathe.

8. To work with the bundle of herbs, start by taking a moment to connect to them. Bring the herbs to your nose, inhale their scent, and give thanks to them for supporting you. Feel their medicine moving through your body. Use the bundle of herbs like a broom to sweep across your body. You may use light touch or firm.

9. Use your breath as a tool to move the energy in your body. Inhale deeply. Exhale and make a sound. Invite your emotions to freely flow through breath and song. Cry. Scream. Sing. If you find you are holding your breath or are breathing shallowly, take a few deep breaths. For the aires to flow, your breath must be moving.

10. Use sacred smoke or a limpia liniment to keep yourself and the space energetically clean.

11. Continue to work until you feel that your process is complete. I know when I am complete when I feel a sense of peace and relief.

12. During the limpia, we open up energetically to give birth to our aires, so it is important to close ourselves after the limpia. We can close ourselves by wrapping ourselves tightly in a blanket. We can also firmly squeeze each puerta/joint. Swaddle yourself and rest.

13. When you are ready to finish the ritual, thank all the energies that were present to support you.

After your limpia is complete, allow yourself time to transition. You may feel a little spacey and altered. I always recommend that my clients don't have anything planned in their schedules after they receive a limpia. It may take a few minutes or hours to transition, depending on the intensity of the process. Fully integrating the process will take a few days or even weeks. Eat a little piece of chocolate and drink hot herbal tea. Clean your space with copal smoke or a limpia liniment. Offer the used herbs and egg back to the earth and give thanks to Tonantzin for receiving your energetic waste. Ask that these energies be transformed into something beautiful.

## Tlazolteotl: Guardian of la Limpia

Elders taught me that whenever a limpia or purification occurred, Tlazolteotl was present.[12]

—Patrisia Gonzales

Mother Earth Tonantzin is a dynamic and living being whose energy and function change with seasons and cycles. In springtime, Tonantzin gives us new life: buds appear on trees, flowers blossom, and green leaves sprout. By winter, the growing cycle of plant life ends. Trees lose their leaves; plants die back or go dormant. All human and animal life also undergoes a similar cycle. We are born, we live and die, and our bodies are received back into the earth. This sacred duality of life and death relates to dual aspects of the earth, the energies of Tlazohteotl and Tlazolteotl.[*]

Tlazohteotl (from the Nahuatl word *tlazohtla*, which is love) loves us and gives us energy for life. Tlazohteotl provides us with all the precious energy we need for life. Tlazohteotl lovingly shelters us, nourishes us, heals us, protects us, and gives us beauty and spiritual sustenance. Its duality, Tlazolteotl (from the Nahuatl word *tlazolli*, which means waste) has the power to remove, destroy, and transform what we no longer need.[13] Tlazolteotl is called Great Mother and She Who Regenerates with Love, and presides over medicinal herbs, pregnancy, labor,

---

[*] Tlazolteotl and Tlazohteotl are very similar words, except for the letters *l* and *h*.

birth, and midwives.[14]* She also is the guardian of the temezcalli, the "house of sweat," which is a sacred space for purification, labor, and birth.** Tlazolteotl was greatly misunderstood and misrepresented by Spanish colonizers, who referred to her as "filth eater" or "goddess of dirt," "witch," and "demon."[15] They mistranslated Tlazolteotl's sacred function of dying, composting, and transformation as something sinful and perverse.

When we become conscious of the energy of Tlazolteotl, we can work with her in our self-limpia practice. (See the Tonantzin meditation in chapter 4.) I always send the energies I release in my self-limpia back to the earth, and I ask permission of the earth to receive these energies. This is why it is a good practice to bury or compost the egg and herbs we use in our limpias.

# Baños

The limpia is only one of many cleansing practices in curanderismo. In this tradition, one of the most important spaces for cleaning ourselves physically, emotionally, and spiritually is in the temescal. When we enter the temescal, we are entering the womb of Tonanztin. Inside the warm, moist darkness, we pray, sing, and rub bundles of fresh herbs over our naked bodies. We release our aires through sweat and tears. Certain curanderas called temescaleras specialize in leading temescal ceremonies.

The temescal is a sacred and sensuous experience. I love being embraced by the darkness and feeling the heat penetrate my skin. I love scrubbing my body with herbs and how their scent mingles with my sweat. Inside the temescal, I have felt my ancestors' pain and have seen flashes of their faces smiling at me in the darkness. I have connected to the wounded little girl inside me and held her while she cried. Inside the sacred womb of the earth, I have felt tenderness

---

* To learn more about Tlazolteotl and more about her connection to pregnancy, birth, and midwives, I highly recommend Patrisia Gonzales's book *Red Medicine: Traditional Indigenous Rites of Birthing and Healing*.

** The temezcalli is often called the "Mexican sweat lodge," yet it is different in both construction and function than sweat lodges of northern Native American Plains tribes such as the Lakota. Traditionally temezcallis are constructed of adobe, whereas many sweat lodges are built with willow. The temezcalli is a sacred space for people who are menstruating, pregnant, or birthing, whereas in sweat lodges there often exist protocols prohibiting people who are menstruating or pregnant from participating.

and love from Tonantzin so powerful it is indescribable. I love coming out of the temescal feeling freshly reborn.

In an ideal world, every community would have its own temescal, and we would all be able to enter the temescal regularly. However, spaces with a temescal are not as commonplace in the United States today as they are in Mexico. As a result, many of us don't have access to a temescal. One of my favorite ways to create a similar ritual for myself is through the practice of baños.

Baños are ritual herbal baths. To do a baño, we make a strong herbal tea and then use it to bathe ourselves. All of the same herbs we use for limpias can be used in baños, although for baños we can use fresh or dried herbs. Sometimes I also incorporate salts into my baños. Here is the way taught to me by Doña Enriqueta and Maestra Estela Román to do a traditional baño. It may be done in a bathtub, shower, or outside if you have privacy.

1. Gather the herbs you will be using. Make your offerings to the plants and ask for their support.
2. Bring a large pot of water to a boil on the stove.
3. Add the herbs to the pot while you focus on your intention and prayers for yourself.
4. Simmer the herbs on low heat for at least twenty minutes.
5. When the herbal water is good and strong, turn off the heat. Let the water cool down enough to be comfortable to the touch.
6. Bring the pot of herbal water to your shower or bath.
7. Use a ladle to slowly pour the warm water over your body. Ask the plantitas and the water for healing. Allow your intuition to guide you to pour the water on the parts of your body where it is needed.
8. When you have finished, dry yourself off. Lie down and wrap yourself in blankets and sheets. Be sure to cover your head. Rest and allow the healing to continue.
9. As you do for a limpia, give yourself time and space to transition. Eating some chocolate and drinking warm herbal tea will help.

Another option is to pour the pot of hot herbs into the bathtub. You may strain out the herbs or pour the entire contents of the pot into your bath. I prefer not to strain the herbs, as I enjoy seeing all my plant friends floating around me while I bathe. I will grab a handful of leaves and rub them on my body. The only disadvantage to not straining out the herbs is that you will have to clean them up. Be sure to have a drain strainer to catch the herbal material so that it doesn't clog your drain. Some curanderx create beautiful healing baths by sprinkling fresh flowers directly into the bath water. Adding the flowers directly to the bath retains their color and vibrancy.

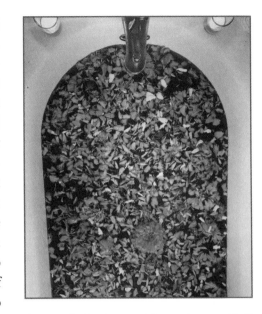

I love taking baths, and I do much of my healing work on myself in the bathtub. I make my baths into a sacred space for tending to myself. I prefer to take baths at night and turn off all the lights, so I am soaking in the peaceful darkness. Feel free to experiment, be creative, and create your own rituals for bathing.

## HERBAL BATH SALT RECIPES

When we bathe with herbs, we are absorbing the healing benefits of the plants through our skin. Baths are particularly beneficial for the skin, muscles, and joints, yet all parts of the body can benefit from an herbal bath. Baths help us relax and unwind and are an excellent way to let go of stress and the aires we may be carrying. We can mix our herbs with salt to create our own herbal bath salt blends. There are many kinds of salt that can be used in baths. Sea salt is a good choice and usually inexpensive. Epsom salts are a great addition to bath salt blends, although they are technically not a salt but a mineral called magnesium sulfate. Epsom salts are an excellent ally to help relieve pain, relax tight muscles, help the body to detoxify, and help with sleep. Himalayan salt is high in trace minerals and adds a nice pink color to your bath salt blends. Sodium bicarbonate (baking soda) also helps with sore muscles, is soothing to the skin, and can help relieve itchy rashes such as those caused by poison oak.

### Heart-Healing Bath

1 cup salt mixture
¼ cup rose petals
¼ cup cempohualxochitl or calendula petals
Optional: flower essences

### Cleansing and Protection Bath

1 cup salt mixture
¼ cup yarrow flowers
¼ cup ruda

### Dreamtime Bath

1 cup salt mixture
¼ cup mugwort
¼ cup rosemary

### Calming Bath

1 cup salt mixture
¼ cup manzanilla
¼ cup lavender

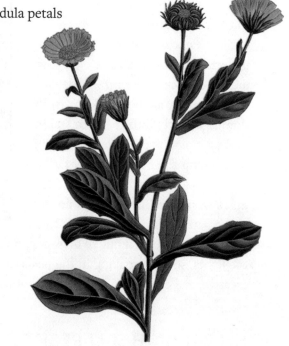

Tending to ourselves with limpias, baños, and other self-care rituals is not just a practice but a lifestyle. We learn to be responsible for our own energy. We learn to recognize when we are out of whack and need to take time with la medicina to rebalance ourselves. We learn to take care of our own aires, instead of allowing them to accumulate for months and years. When we face challenges and difficulties in our lives, we are empowered with practices that help us be more resilient. The ancestors of this tradition carefully stewarded these practices through generations so that they would be available for us. As we make these practices part of our own lives, we ensure that nuestra medicina will continue to thrive and be available for future generations.

# SPOTLIGHT

## Alejandra Olguin
### (she/her/ella)

> "When we're doing limpias, we're midwifing the aires. We're helping release those aires, and there's a transformation in every single limpia. It's an opportunity to release something old and renew yourself. [Each time, we] come out of it a little bit different. Birth offers release and renewal too, but you birth a baby instead of an aire."

Alejandra was born in Napa Valley to parents from the Mixteca region of Oaxaca, Mexico. She grew up visiting her grandparents and extended family in Oaxaca every summer, and first experienced her ancestral medicine through her abuelas, one of whom would heal susto with tobacco smoke. Alejandra is a clinical social worker, traditional birthworker, promotora of curanderismo, and cofounder of Nueva Luz (re)Birth and Family Care. I first met her as my student, but I consider her a trusted friend and colleague. Alejandra embodies strength and sweetness and a heartfelt dedication to community healing.

### ALEJANDRA OLGUIN SPEAKS:

I grew up losing the medicine for a big part of my life. My mom would clean us with the egg, which I didn't really understand as a kid. But once we got older, I don't remember her doing limpias anymore. The more my family became involved in the church, the more they rejected our ancestral medicine. They would say, "No son cosas de Dios."

In my twenties I started going to Oaxaca by myself, and that's when I started my process of understanding who I was, where I came from, and feeling a sense of pride around it. I started going back with a different mindset, started to develop my own identity, finally finding a sense of belonging. Spirit was calling me, and I wanted to reconnect to the land and to know more about our family medicine. I started spending a lot of time with my grandparents and asked them a lot of

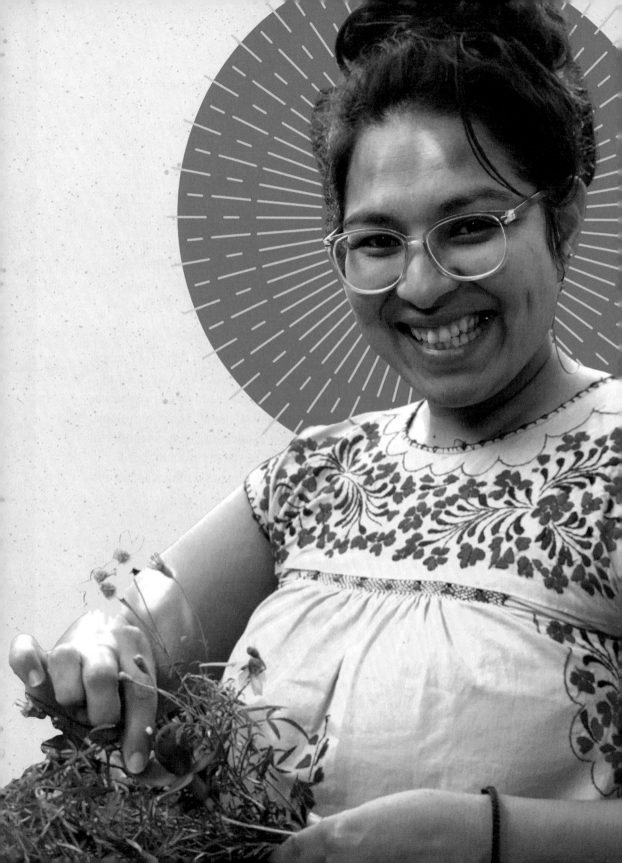

questions about what it was like when they were young, growing up in our pueblo.

A friend in Oaxaca told me she was going to get a limpia, and I said, "What's that? I want to come. I want a limpia!" It was a powerful experience and it sparked something in me, and I wanted to learn more.

I started getting interested in birthwork, and I interviewed my grandma because she birthed all nine kids at home with a midwife. She gave me this whole list of herbs she would use for the postpartum bath. She told me about her birth story, about the temescal and cerradas. It was so exciting to learn that my grandmother knew this stuff! At that time, I was searching everywhere else because I had a sense that she wasn't connected to the medicine anymore because she was so Catholic. But when it came to talking about remedios, she was very open about it.

My mom had a traumatic birth story. She was alone, and she didn't speak the language. What if my mom had stayed in her community? I wanted to know what happens to ancestral birthing practices when people emigrate. In my thesis, I highlighted stories of immigrant women who are the first generation to birth in the US. I also wanted to talk to women who were changing the birthing narrative and reclaiming the ancestral practices of birthing and really holding birth as a ceremony again.

In my work, I started realizing how similar it felt when I was doing a limpia and when I was at a birth and holding space for someone in that process of releasing. In a limpia, you're holding space for somebody to encounter that pain they have inside, and you hold that space so that they can release it. But in order to release it, they have to feel really safe. You guide them and help them open up. And when they finally release, when they cry or when that release happens, it's so exciting.

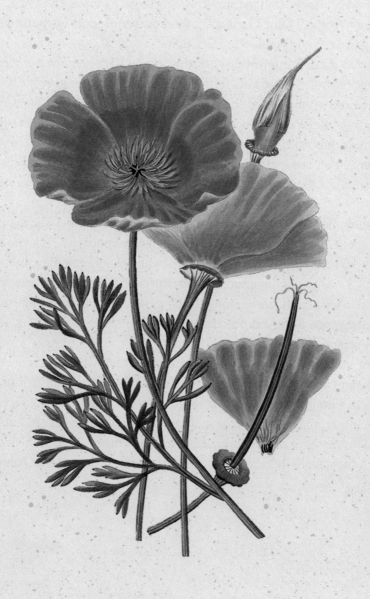

# CHAPTER 13

# La Medicina of Dreams

On this fearless path of the dreamer, you will recover the brilliance that is normally beyond your reach and out of view: you've actually decided to become awake within the great dream. You will recognize that waking life is the dream; and dreaming is the time where real decisions are made, where the eyes witness the eternal light of life.[1]

—Eleanor Barron-Druckrey

Learning to value our dreams is a step toward decolonizing our way of gaining knowledge. We are trained in contemporary American culture to believe that knowledge is something we need to obtain from a source outside ourselves, and often at a steep price. Knowledge isn't seen as something gained by life experience, but something that we are entitled to because we have paid a high price for it.

Our dreams offer us an opportunity to shift into a new paradigm of coming into knowledge. What would it look like if everyone, regardless of their age, race, gender identity, religion, or class, had equal access to a source of wisdom? What if everyone had an equal opportunity to tap into a source of knowledge that comes directly from our ancestors and from the infinite archives of the cosmos? What if we all were trained to access the healing knowledge that is inside all of us? What if this wisdom were free and available to all? By working with and honoring our dreams, we have the chance to center our access to wisdom, guidance, and healing inside ourselves. As we build relationship with our dreams, we learn how to work with them to empower ourselves.

## Dream Traditions of Ancient Mexico

Dreams played a fundamental role in the traditions of ancient Mexico. According to more than five thousand years of oral tradition, the ancient cultures of Mexico, including the Olmecs, Chichimecas, Xochicalcas, Mexicas, and Toltecs, all had developed highly sophisticated systems of dreaming. In fact, the name

Mexico comes from two Nahuatl words, *metzli* (moon) and *xictli* (navel), and can be translated as "place of the navel of the moon." The moon presides over the realm of dreams, so another translation of *Mexico* could be "land of the dreamers."[2]

The energetic body that rules the dream state is called the nahual, and our waking state is ruled by the tonal. (The tonal and nahual are discussed in more depth in chapter 10.) When we are awake, our tonal presides around our head, and the nahual rests at the navel. When we go to sleep, the tonal and nahual switch places. The tonal moves down to the navel, and the nahual moves up near the head. With practice, we can train our tonal and nahual to come together near the heart center while we are sleeping. When tonal and nahual unite, they create a new energetic body and a state of consciousness called *temixoch*, which translates to "flowering dreams" and refers to the state of lucid dreaming. Lucid dreaming means we are dreaming (nahual), but "awake" (tonal) in the dream.[3]

In Mexica and Toltec dreaming traditions, it is believed that all the nature of "reality," or that which we experience in our waking lives/tonal state, is first seeded in our dreams. In the fertile darkness of our dreams, our nahual plants the seeds that in turn flower into creations in our waking lives. This means that by learning to shape our dreams, we can also influence and change the waking state of our lives. This practice is called Mexicatzin, which refers to the discipline of gaining conscious control over one's dreams.[4] Mexicatzin involves many exercises, including recapitulation, working with the obsidian mirror, and practicing certain breathing exercises before going to sleep.

## Sacred Sleep

Because of the importance of dreaming in curanderismo, the work of a curanderx does not end when they go to sleep at night. In fact, we have the opportunity to engage in some of our most important work during our sleep and dreamtime. Many people don't think about it, but we spend about a third of our life sleeping, and by the time we are thirty years old, we have been asleep for ten years!

One important function of sleep is to give our physical bodies time to rest and repair. Good sleep is essential to good health. An ideal amount of sleep for an adult is about seven to eight hours per night, but many people regularly receive much less. Lack of sleep can make us feel tired, spacey, and irritable and makes us more vulnerable to disease.

Our busy mainstream culture does not value sleep or rest. We don't listen to our bodies when they feel tired. We simply drink another cup of coffee and eat something sugary to give us a false sense of energy. We ignore our body and power on. We are taught to see rest as "lazy" and downtime as "unproductive."

Many factors can adversely affect our ability to sleep, including physical pain, digestive discomforts, hormonal imbalances, anxiety, depression, and stress. Our sleep is also impacted by external factors, such as caffeine or other stimulants or exercising too late in the day. The quality of light (especially blue light from electronics), sound, and temperature in our bedroom also can impact our sleep.

# Herbal Allies for Sleep and Dreams

To support sleep, take herbs in a tea or tincture about an hour before bed. If staying asleep is a challenge, keep herbs near your bed so that you can easily take another dose if you wake up.

To work with herbs for dreams, you may take them as a tea, tincture, baño, mister, or flower essence, or place them in a dream pillow.

## Scullcap
*Scutellaria lateriflora*

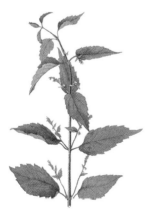

Scullcap is in the mint family and fairly easy to grow. It prefers partial shade. The best time to harvest scullcap for medicine is when it is flowering. The best tincture is made from the fresh leaves and flowers.

As an herbal nervine, scullcap relaxes hot, frazzled nerves. It has been used traditionally to treat spasms, nerve pain, restlessness, irritability, nervous exhaustion, headaches, insomnia, anxiety, and phobias. It helps our bodies release tension when we feel wound up. Scullcap is a good herbal ally for sleep disrupted by emotional distress. It can help ease mind chatter and soothe emotions that keep us awake. After a long bout with insomnia, I have used scullcap to improve my sleep for the past three decades.

## SUGGESTIONS FOR USE

For adults, take one cup of tea or fifteen to sixty drops of the tincture.

# Passiflora/Passionflower/Tzitzintlápatl
*Passiflora incarnata*

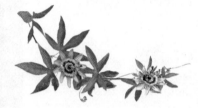

Passionflower is native to many temperate regions of the world, including parts of Mexico and the Southwest, and grows easily in Huchiun/the Bay Area. It is a robust vine with stunningly beautiful flowers that are well loved by bees and other pollinators. It prefers full sun and can be propagated by seeds, cuttings, or root division.

Passionflower relaxes tight, tense muscles. It can relax the physical tension in our bodies that keeps us awake. It relieves restless leg syndrome, temporal mandibular joint (TMJ) disorder, headaches, and back pain. Passionflower quiets racing thoughts that may interfere with sleep. In large doses, it can be sedating, which can help us fall asleep.

## SUGGESTIONS FOR USE

For adults, take one cup of tea or fifteen to sixty drops of the tincture. Passion-flower combines well with scullcap. I recommend trying a tea using equal parts of each herb.

# California Poppy

*Eschscholzia californica*

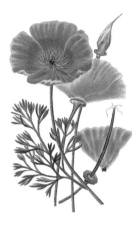

California poppy is not only the California state flower but also a medicinal herb that helps with sleep. California poppy, *Eschscholzia californica*, should not be confused with the opium poppy, *Papaver somniferum*. They are botanically related, but are different plants with different properties. Both plants are relaxing, but California poppy does not contain opiates and is safe and nonaddictive.

California poppy is a protected plant in the state, and you may be fined if you harvest from public spaces. As a native plant, it is acclimated to our climate and soil conditions and easy to grow in most areas of California. It is drought tolerant and needs only light watering in its early stages of growth. Sow the seeds directly into the soil in the late fall or early spring.[5] All parts—the flowers, leaves, stems, and roots—are medicinal, and the poppy is best harvested when in full bloom.

As a sleep aid, California poppy can knock us out. It helps us unwind when we're overstimulated from activity, stress, or caffeine. It calms children who are tired and wired and also helps with sleep disturbed by physical pain. It also increases sleep latency, which is the length of time people stay asleep.

## SUGGESTIONS FOR USE

For adults, take a cup of tea or fifteen to sixty drops of the tincture. Higher doses are more sedating.

## CONTRAINDICATIONS

Do not ingest and drive or do anything that requires quick reflexes and an alert state.

## Other Allies

Many herbs (such as the ones listed previously) help us relax our bodies and minds to promote good sleep. Other herbs, called oneirogens, are helpful for dreamwork, as they can influence our dreams and help with dream recall.

- **Estafiate/mugwort** is a well-known oneirogen that improves dream recall and helps us dream more vividly. However, sometimes its effect is overpowering and causes people to dream so intensely that in the morning they wake up feeling exhausted. Curiously, I have also noticed that for people who are already vivid dreamers, mugwort can have the opposite effect and actually inhibit dreams.
- **Manzanilla** treats insomnia caused by digestive discomforts and helps ease fear and anxiety that may keep us awake. It is my top choice for alleviating nightmares in both children and adults. Manzanilla has a special ability to bring about healing dreams, and I recommend dreaming with it when facing any health challenge.
- **Rosemary/romero** helps us remember our dreams and brings protection in the dream state.
- **The Grandmother Plant** (*Tagetes lemmonii*) has the special ability to activate ancestral dreams. It also brings dreams of healing and guidance.
- **Pericón** is an oneirogen that helps activate vivid and lucid dreams.
- Both **yarrow** and **ruda** provide protection in our dream state.

# Dreaming with Plants

As both an herbalist and a dreamer, I have had a lot of fun exploring the intersection between the dream world and the plant world. In Toltec/Mexica dream traditions, it is believed that everything dreams, including the earth, the animals, the stars, the sun, and the moon. Everything has both a waking-state self (tonal) and a dreaming-state self (nahual). When we dream of plants, we are encountering their nahual. The different nahuales of plants serve different functions in the dream state. For example, l learned that by making offerings to certain plants in the waking state, they will then serve as my protectors in the dream state. I also learned that in our dreams, a plant might not look like plant! The nahual of a plant can shape-shift into any form, and plants can appear in dreams in human or animal form.

Plants influence our dream state. In the waking state, each plant has unique healing qualities and also has different healing qualities in the dream state. We can learn more about plants by dreaming with them. Plants have revealed to me in dreams things about themselves that I never could have learned in books.

Here are some suggestions on how to dream with the plants:

- Place a bit of the herb near where you sleep.
- If it is not contraindicated, take some of the herb before going to sleep, or use it topically or in a bath.
- Incubate a dream with your plant. Before going to sleep, set an intention before bed to dream of this certain herb.
- Pay close attention to which plants show up in your dreams. They may be your special allies.
- If you dream of an herb, take time to learn about its properties, or incorporate it into your life.

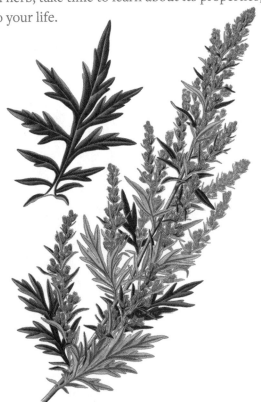

# HERBAL RECIPES FOR SLEEP AND DREAMS

### Healing Dreams

> 1 part manzanilla
> ½ part lavender
> Pinch of rose petals

### Ancestral Dreams

> 1 part Grandmother Plant (*Tagetes lemmonii* )
> 1 part romero
> ½ part yarrow

### Deep Rest

> 1 part scullcap
> 1 part passionflower
> ½ part California poppy

### Dream Activator

> 1 part estafiate
> 1 part pericón
> 1 part romero

### Dream Pillow Blend

> 1 part estafiate
> 1 part manzanilla
> 1 part rosemary
> 1 part lavender

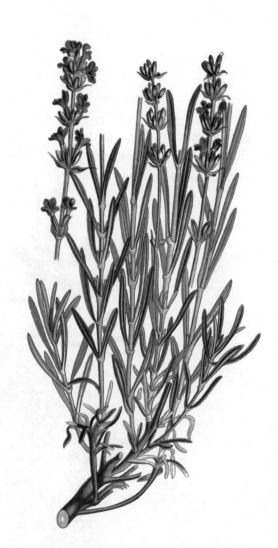

# Dream Journaling

To cultivate our gifts as dreamers, we must first develop a practice of remembering and recording our dreams. Everyone dreams each night, but many of us struggle to remember our dreams. Many factors interfere with dream recall, including stress, past trauma, lack of sleep, and certain medications. Some of these issues can be resolved with lifestyle changes. Often dream recall can improve with the introduction of certain practices, as I will outline. Herbs such as romero can also support dream recall.

An essential step in developing our dream practice is to start keeping a dream journal. This helps us remember and track the messages sent from our dream body or nahual. We must become familiar with our dream landscape and the common themes and patterns in our dreams. When we become intimately acquainted with our dreams, we gain a deeper understanding of ourselves.

## DREAM JOURNALING PRACTICE

1. Keep a journal, pen, and soft light near your bed to write down your dreams.
2. When you wake up, try to stay still and not change your position. Keep your eyes closed and review your dreams.
3. Write down your dreams immediately before getting out of bed.
4. Give each dream a title. This helps you browse back easily though your dream journal and find certain dreams.
5. Other ways to dream journal include drawing, poetry, and audio recordings.

# Dream Incubation

If we are not taught how to work with our dreams, we may be only passive participants with our dream world. We receive dreams, but do not actively engage in calling forth what kinds of dreams may come.

To learn how to incubate dreams is to learn how to be an active participant with our dreams. Dream incubation is the practice of creating space and setting intention for certain dreams to come. In the Mexica tradition, the practice is called "planting dreams."

There is no one way to incubate a dream. Dream incubation is about creating space, setting intention, and saying prayers for particular dreams to come. Each dreamer will bring their own spiritual and cultural practices to the way they incubate their dreams. I will offer some general suggestions, but I encourage you to listen to your own intuition and guidance about what is best for you.

## DREAM INCUBATION PRACTICE

1. Set your dream intention and write down your intention in your dream journal.
2. Create a sacred space for dreaming.
3. Take time to pray or meditate before going to sleep.
4. As you are falling asleep, repeat your intention in your mind.
5. If you wake up in the night, bring your intention back to mind.
6. Record the dreams that come.
7. For the most effective dream incubation, I recommend repeating this practice for at least four nights in a row.

Don't be upset if the answer to your incubation doesn't come right away. Dreams have their own timing. Sometimes the answer to my incubation comes days, weeks, or months later.*

# Honoring Dreams

We respectfully interact with our medicine dreams by acknowledging and thanking the energies that delivered the dream. I have been taught to honor the spirits of the dream by making an offering. This is basic spiritual etiquette, to give

---

* When you incubate a dream, if you are sleeping next to another person, don't be surprised if they catch your dream! This happened once with me and my partner. I was incubating a dream, but didn't recall any dreams when I woke up. My partner said to me, "I had the most unusual dream." She went on to describe her dream, and it seemed to be an answer to my dream incubation question. Perhaps the dream GPS navigated to our bed but arrived at my partner's dream space instead!

thanks for the gift that has been given. If we don't thank the spirits of our dreams, then perhaps they will think we don't appreciate their offerings and will stop working with us. If I don't make a physical offering, I will simply say a prayer of thanks. Finding a way to engage with the dream is also a way of honoring the dream. Each of us will do this in a different way, and each dream may require a different action to honor it.

WAYS TO HONOR YOUR DREAMS

- Write down your dream, and journal your thoughts and feelings about it.
- Creatively engage with your dream through art, poetry, or music.
- Meditate on your dream.
- Share your dream with others.
- Bring a representation of your dream into your waking life. For example, if you dream of an ancestor, put their image or name on your altar.
- Take action to honor the dream. When I had a series of dreams about wolves, I found an organization that protected endangered wolves, and made a donation.

# The Symbolic Language of Dreams

The language of dreams is much different than spoken word. Dreams are often not rational or logical. Instead, dreams speak in a mysterious language of symbols, colors, riddles, and puns. The Mexica/Toltec dream traditions pay much attention to the movement, directionality, and size of the dream symbols and objects. Many symbols that appear in dreams are universal, which means that they have similar meaning for different people around the world.

Many of us try to understand our dreams with our rational mind. However, the messages of dreams are often best unlocked by engaging the creative and intuitive part of our brain. Although writing down my dreams is an important practice, I find that the energy of my dream seems to fizzle when I put it into written English. When instead I take the time to draw or sketch my dream, I am able to preserve more of its magic.

Every part of the dream is a symbol whose meaning we can unpack. We can work with the symbols by drawing them, meditating on them, and allowing ourselves to freely associate about the symbol. We can also work with the symbols through sound and movement. Although we can explore each symbol of any dream, I normally work with the symbols that are the most charged or most compelling for me.

The understanding of our dreams takes both effort and time. Each dream and each dream symbol has multiple levels and multiple meanings. Listening to our dreams requires both patience and a willingness to hang out in the unknown. In my life, some of my dreams are like stories that I return to time after time. Each time I revisit these dreams, they reveal something else to me about myself, my life, and about the great mystery of the universe.

## Doorway to Our Underworlds

In the Mexica and Toltec dream traditions, dreams are seen as an entryway to the nine underworlds. Here all of our shadows lurk: our buried emotions, our fears, our negative repetitive patterns, our ancestral patterns, and our addictions. When we pay attention to our dreams, they may reveal to us things about ourselves that we may not be able to recognize. They may reveal parts of ourselves that we don't like and want to reject. My dreams have made me face all of my aires in a way that is uncomfortable but that eventually helps me grow and evolve as a person. We can choose to ignore our underworlds, but ultimately they control us until we deal with them.

## Source of Guidance

Our dreams can also be gifts of healing, support, creativity, and spiritual development. This aspect of dreams helps balance out all our harrowing encounters with our underworlds. We can work with our dreams to help us make choices in our lives. Often when I am about to make a big decision, I allow myself some time to dream on it. I have taken many big steps in my life based on the guidance of my dreams.

We can also meet and connect to our spirit guides in our dreams. How do we know when we encounter a spirit guide? The dream may have a particular quality of energy, like the buzz of electricity. The dream may convey a special feeling, like the fluttering of our heart when we fall in love. The dream may come in extraordinary detail of color, shape, and sound. Or we may wake up just knowing that we had a spiritual encounter. Our dream guides can take many forms—a person, an animal, or a magical creature. They may communicate with language, or they may convey their messages to us nonverbally. The same being may appear repeatedly in our dreams, and over time we start to recognize them as our spirit guide.

It takes work, patience, and time to develop our relationship to our dream guides. If we acknowledge the dreams, our guides know that we are present and listening. If we ignore their messages, our guides may decide to stop sending them to us. Give yourself time to contemplate your dreams and find a way to honor the messages you have received.

# Healing Dreams

Our dreams can be rich sources of healing for our bodies, minds, and emotions. Dreams can also help us heal and resolve our relationships, even with people who are no longer in our lives or who are no longer alive. Healing dreams can occur in different ways. We can receive direct healing in a dream. In some dreams, a person, animal, magical creature, or plant may appear and perform a healing on us.

Our body speaks to us in our dreams, and we need to learn how to listen and decode its messages. We can receive clues to our health challenges, including issues that may be root causes. Dreams may also offer us advice on what we need to do in waking life to resolve our health challenges, such as what foods to eat or herbs to take. For people facing terminal diagnoses, dreams can also help them prepare for the transition of death.

# Ancestral Dreams

Dreams can be doorways to other times and other dimensions. We can travel in dreams to the future or to the past. Dreams are a borderland where the living can encounter those who have died. It is not uncommon when people die for them to make an appearance soon thereafter in the dreams of their loved ones. Sometimes family members will be alerted to the death of a loved one through a dream.

# RaheNi's Dream Story

When I was sixteen and staying with the only person in my blood family who fully accepted me as queer, I had a female friend (not a lover) spend the night. My abuela, who lived upstairs, saw her leave in the morning and assumed that something sexual had occurred in my room. My abuela proceeded to go into the room, lit white candles, and began to pray to Jesus to remove "the devil" from the space. I was so angered and deeply hurt. After that, I didn't engage with her much until she was on her deathbed, and then all she could do was cry. Many years later, my abuela came to me in a vision, and the first thing she said was, "I'm sorry for what I did. I'm sorry I didn't understand who you were. I know now that you are a beautiful person." And we talked there in the spirit realm, and it was such a healing experience.

This was validation that when we cross over, if we were generally "good people" doing our best in this world, we are given divine all-knowing vision, and that vision is free of colonized thinking and full of love and acceptance. Your ancestors, those wise ones, those good-hearted ones, they love you, they see you, and they are grateful for you. Yes, you who are queer, you who are two-spirit, you who may seem "different." YOU ARE SACRED . . . YOU ARE LOVED!!! Do not be afraid to show your true self to your ancestors!

According to the Toltec/Mexica dreaming traditions, the north direction relates to the ancestors. In dreams, the direction we are facing is considered north. Ancestors may appear from the north or may come in the shape of a dog (which relates to ancestors), or they can appear as a luminescent energy or light. I have found that ancestral visitations in dreams are often accompanied by strong emotions, as though I am being reunited with a long-lost friend. Prayers, intentions, and plant medicine can also activate our ancestral dreams.

# Collective Dreaming

But regardless of the suffering, the dreamers, the great messengers, will show you lasting truths to help you travel through this dim, dismal period.[6]

—Eleanor Barron-Druckrey

Our dreams are intimate, personal, and sacred. Oftentimes it is important to keep our dreams to ourselves, as they can reveal our vulnerabilities, our hidden emotions, and all that is buried in our unconscious. Our dream world, the realm of the nahual, is also a part of our spiritual power, which must be protected. It is important to exercise discretion when sharing dreams and, when you do share, to always keep part of the dream private. But we can benefit from sharing our dreams with others. Dream sharing is a part of many traditional Indigenous cultures, where dreams are often a source of prophecy, healing, and spiritual guidance. The foundation of Tenochtitlan (today Mexico City, Mexico) originated in a dream. The Mexica people, during their journey of hundreds of years from Aztlan to Tenochtitlan, were guided by a hummingbird that appeared in a dream.

Sharing dreams with other people can be a powerful way to access the wisdom and magic of our dreams. When we share dreams, we tap into the mystery of the collective dream. We can observe the patterns and symbols that weave through one another's dreams and humbly realize that we are part of a much greater force that is dreaming through us. We can receive guidance from dreams even when they are not our own.

Some of the most powerful lessons I have received from dreamtime have come from other people's dreams. Sharing dreams also allows for the gifted dreamers in our communities to emerge. These people have an extraordinary talent for dreaming and may often dream prophetically. When they are given the space to share their dreams, the dreams may contain messages for the entire community.

We can also practice dreaming together as a collective. On overnight field trips, my students and I have dreamed together to connect to the spirit of the land and ask what the land needed of us. We have also dreamed collectively with certain plants to learn more about their medicine. We can dream collectively to petition for healing and guidance for our communities and for the world. The possibilities of collective dreaming are endless.

# Final Thoughts on Dreaming

Due to colonization, industrialization, and other oppressive forces, many people have lost touch with the power of nighttime and the medicine of their dreams. Yet in many traditional cultures, dreams have always played an important role in maintaining the well-being of both individuals and communities. When we are disconnected from our dreams, we are disconnected from our personal medicine and power. When we no longer honor the messages received by dreamers in our communities, we all suffer the consequences. Dreamers receive important messages from the spiritual and ancestral realms that can guide us collectively during this challenging time if we just create space to listen to them. The world urgently needs its dreamers to guide us through this challenging time on earth in which our very existence as a species is endangered.

As I noted earlier, in the Mexica/Toltec tradition, it is believed that everything dreams. The plants, animals, rocks, earth, moon, sun, stars, and planets all dream; all have a nahual. Each night when we sleep, we have an extraordinary opportunity to interact with the dreams of the universe. Although some people may have exceptional dreaming talent, all of us have the capability to develop themselves as a dreamer. Dreams are part of everyone's ancestral medicine, and they are an essential part of the curanderx toolkit. My prayer and intention are that you will be inspired to work with your dreams to help heal yourself and to tap into the vast resource of dreamtime. As we grow stronger as individual dreamers, may we also learn to apply our skills to dream for the collective and guide us through this difficult transition on earth.

.

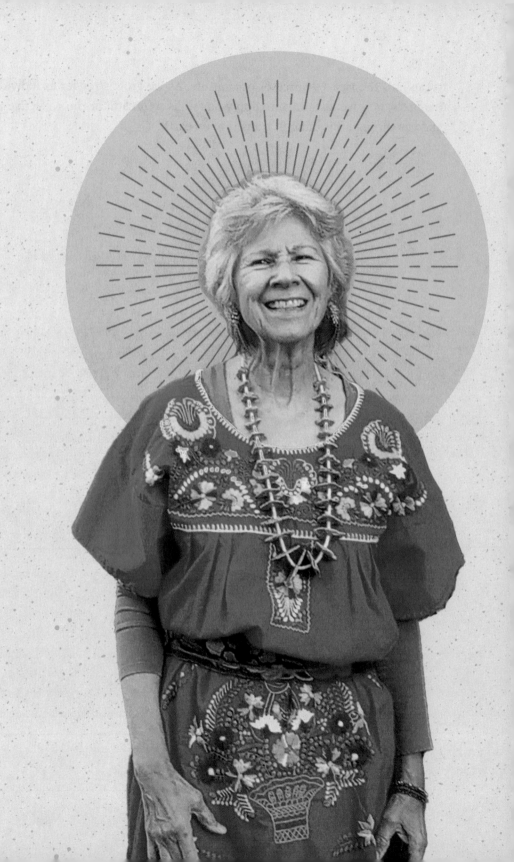

# SPOTLIGHT

# Eleanor "Ellie" Barron-Druckrey
## (she/her/ella)

> "My message to the world would be simple: As the ancestors would say, our dreams are the seat of reality; the waking state is the dream! There is only Spirit. The aires are the dream from which we must awaken. Waking up in our dreams is the only task assigned while we are here on earth."

Eleanor Barron-Druckrey is a curandera of dreams. She has dedicated her life to remembering her ancestral dreaming practices. She was born to Mexican immigrants in Southern California/Tongva territory, grew up in the Central Valley/Yokuts territory, and moved to the Bay Area/Ohlone and Miwok territory as a young adult. Ellie is the author of two books on dreaming, *Corn Woman Sings: A Medicine Woman's Dream Map* and *A Dream Map to the Sixth Sun*. When I first met Ellie at a curanderismo workshop in Sacramento/Nisenan territory, I had been working with my own dreams for decades and suspected that dreams played an important role in our traditional medicine. However, Ellie was the first person I met who gave specific teachings on dreams from a Mexican cultural perspective. I was thrilled to meet her, and she became my maestra, friend, and a regular teacher in the Curanderx Toolkit class.

Ellie was raised in a fundamentalist Christian home and had no sense of curanderismo as a young person. Her father's dream world provided the one connection to her Mexican culture of healing: "My father was a dreamer and would always talk about his dreams. I started dreaming really early in my life, maybe age five or six or even younger when I started bringing my dreams to the table."

As a university student in the 1970s and 1980s, Ellie didn't receive support for her interest in dreams and Mexican traditional medicine, even in her Chicano studies classes. After college, she started a daily practice of writing her dreams down. Quickly, her dreams provided her the guidance she had been seeking in waking life. As she explained, in her dreams, "My meeting with the ancestors started happening immediately." Ellie met a dream guide whom she called Grandmother.

## ELLIE BARRON-DRUCKREY SPEAKS:

My greatest challenges have come from internalized colonization. Many of my life choices were a result of the trauma of being a person of color in this country and the impact of racism, poverty, and the push to consider science more valid and important than creativity. I definitely feel that my struggles through school were a result of the influence to ignore the heart, the feminine, mysticism, and creativity.

But then I met a woman who invited herself on my journey. She didn't say anything to me; she just said, "Can I come with you?" And I said, "Yes, of course." And she became Grandmother. Eventually she would show up in my dreams, and when she showed up, there was always this illumination around her that pulled my heartstrings to her. And she began to speak to me. She began to train me.

If I had that wisdom and knowledge within my dreams, then, surely, I thought, everybody else did too; their healing would be mine and mine theirs. Dreaming opened me up to my destiny, and I wanted to share that with others. It has not been a straight line, and slowly, something has been happening where I am able to teach people to turn inward and together look at the benefits of following the advice of the Ancestors.

Our Ancestors—and I might add that this is the greatest challenge for us today—believed that the waking state was "the dream," and our spiritual reality—our dreamtime—reality. It's taken me my seventy-seven years in this realm to fully comprehend that spirituality is more vital and necessary than the chaos and confusion of the waking state. Love, compassion, and forgiveness are truly the path of transformation. And, I might add, the only way to happiness and peace.

In the past, I've encouraged my students to awaken within their dreams; to make conscious decisions and thereby expand the consciousness of their dreams into the waking state. Now, I encourage them to work with the aires in their waking state and transcend their negative emotions by living from Spirit. Both approaches are difficult.

# Notes

**CHAPTER 1: SEEDS**

1. Elena Avila with Joy Parker, *Woman Who Glows in the Dark: A Curandera Reveals Traditional Aztec Secrets of Physical and Spiritual Health* (New York: J. P. Tarcher/Putnam, 1999), 39.
2. Patrisia Gonzales, *Red Medicine: Traditional Indigenous Rites of Birthing and Healing* (Tucson: University of Arizona Press, 2012).
3. Cheo Torres, personal interview with the author, January 13, 2020.
4. Avila, 84.
5. Maria Miranda, personal interview with the author, June 23, 2021.
6. Berenice Dimas, written interview with the author, June 26, 2021.
7. Avila, 19.
8. Avila, 28.
9. Avila, 28.

**CHAPTER 2: ROOTS AND FLOWERS**

1. María Margarita Návar, *Mujer zapoteca de las nubes: La vida de la partera-curandera Enriqueta Contreras Contreras; Zapotec Woman of the Clouds: The Life of the Midwife-Healer Enriqueta Contreras Contreras* (Austin, TX: Zapotec Press, 2010).
2. Joie Davidow, *Infusions of Healing: A Treasury of Mexican-American Herbal Remedies* (New York: Simon & Schuster, 1999), 20–21.
3. Eliseo "Cheo" Torres, "Mexican Folk Medicine and Folk Beliefs," PowerPoint presentation from Traditional Medicine without Borders class, University of New Mexico, Albuquerque, 2004, http://www.unm.edu/~cheo/LONG.pdf.
4. *The Burning Times,* directed by Donna Read, written by Erna Biffie (National Film Board of Canada, 1990).
5. Maria Miranda, personal interview with the author, June 23, 2021.
6. Max Dashu, "Witch Hunts," n.d., https://www.suppressedhistories.net/catalog/witchhunts.html; "Police Seize Elderly Mexican Man over 'Witch' Killing," CNN World, November 13, 2009, http://edition.cnn.com/2009

/WORLD/americas/11/13/mexico.witchcraft.killing/; Victoria Baena, "The Murder of a Witch," *Dissent*, Fall 2020, https://www.dissentmagazine.org/article/the-murder-of-a-witch.

7. Gonzales, chap. 1.
8. Gonzales, chap. 1.
9. Avila, 15.
10. Jesus C. Villa, "African Healing in Mexican Curanderismo" (master's thesis, Arizona State University, 2016), 46.
11. Villa, 44.
12. Villa, 44.
13. Villa, 38–47.
14. Villa, 45.
15. Villa, 46.
16. Herman L. Bennett, *Colonial Blackness: A History of Afro-Mexico* (Bloomington: Indiana University Press, 2009), 18–19.
17. Villa, 70.
18. Villa, 63.
19. Villa, 64.
20. Alejandra Olguin, personal interview with the author, August 25, 2019.
21. Maria Miranda, personal interview with the author, June 23, 2021.
22. Eleanor Barron-Druckrey, personal interview with the author, April 3, 2019.
23. Jennie Marie Luna, *Danza Mexica: Indigenous Identity, Spirituality, Activism, and Performance* (PhD diss., UC Davis, 2011), 159.
24. Lorena Valdivia Márquez, *Sacramento en el Movimiento: Chicano Politics in the Civil Rights Era* (PhD diss., UC San Diego, 2010), 225–305.
25. Dixie Reid, "Historical Collection Shows Impact Sac State Activists Had on Chicano Movement," Sacramento State Newsroom, February 19, 2021, https://www.csus.edu/news/newsroom/stories/2021/2/chicano-history.html.
26. Luna, 169.
27. Mujeres de Maiz (Women of the Corn), https://www.mujeresdemaiz.com.

## CHAPTER 3: REMEMBERING ANCESTRAL WAYS OF WELLNESS

1. Anna Joyce, *The Sixth Sun: The Spiritual Path and Practice of Mexican-American Curanderismo* (PhD diss., California Institute of Integral Studies, San Francisco, 2011), 405.

2. Patricia Chicueyi Coatl, personal email correspondence with the author, February 2021.

## CHAPTER 4: SELF-CARE IS A REVOLUTIONARY ACT

1. Audre Lorde, "A Burst of Light: Living with Cancer," in *A Burst of Light and Other Essays* (New York: Courier Dover Publications, 2017), 130.
2. Resmaa Menakem, *My Grandmother's Hands: Racialized Trauma and the Pathway to Mending Our Hearts and Bodies* (Las Vegas, NV: Central Recovery Press), 2017.
3. Anna Joyce, *The Sixth Sun: The Spiritual Path and Practice of Mexican-American Curanderismo* (PhD diss., California Institute of Integral Studies, San Francisco, 2011), 288.

## CHAPTER 5: CREATING SACRED SPACE

1. Patricia Chicueyi Coatl, "Nauhcampa: Los Cuatro Rumbos" (pamphlet for Calpulli Huey Papalotl, n.d.), 4.
2. Jennie Marie Luna, *Danza Mexica: Indigenous Identity, Spirituality, Activism, and Performance* (PhD diss., UC Davis, 2011), 343.
3. Patricia Chicueyi Coatl, "The Four Basic Elements of the Momoxtli," *Calmecac Huey Papalotl* (unpublished class reader, 2014), 70.
4. Luna, 342.
5. Sergio Magaña (Ocelocoyotl), 2012–2021—*The Dawn of the Sixth Sun: The Path of Quetzalcoatl* (Giaveno, Italy: BlossomingBooks, 2012), 5.
6. Magaña, 151.
7. Leonardo López Luján y Alfredo López Austin, "Las cihuateteo contraatacan. El glifo 1 mono del Centro Histórico de la Ciudad de México," *Arqueología Mexicana*, no. 152 (Julio/Agosto 2018): 80–83.
8. Magaña, 57.
9. Notes from The Four Waters and the Four Fires, class taught by Sergio Magaña (Ocelocoyotl), September 3–4, 2016, Ashland, Oregon.

## CHAPTER 6: HERBAL ALLIES

1. Robin Wall Kimmerer, *Braiding Sweetgrass: Indigenous Wisdom, Scientific Knowledge, and the Teachings of Plants* (Minneapolis, MN: Milkweed Editions, 2013), 128.

2. Stefano Mancuso, *Brilliant Green: The Surprising History and Science of Plant Intelligence*, trans. Joan Benham (Washington, DC: Island Press, 2016), 40.

3. Estela Román, "Lo frio y lo caliente, energía kin-fuerza vital," Zoom class, May 2020; Alfredo López Austin, *Textos de medicina náhuatl, Cuarto edición* (Ciudad de México: Instituto de Investigaciones Históricas, Universidad Nacional Autonoma de México, 1993), 16–22.

4. López Austin, *Textos de medicina náhuatl*, 16–22.

5. Román, "Lo frio y lo caliente."

6. Eliseo "Cheo" Torres, *Healing with Herbs and Rituals: A Mexican Tradition* (Albuquerque: University of New Mexico Press, 2006), 86.

7. Jassem G. Mahdi, "Medicinal Potential of Willow: A Chemical Perspective of Aspirin Discovery," *Journal of Saudi Chemical Society* 14, no. 3 (July 2010): 317–22.

8. Veronika Butterweck, "Mechanism of Action of St John's Wort in Depression: What Is Known?" *CNS Drugs* 17, no. 8 (2003): 539–62. https://doi.org/10.2165/00023210-200317080-00001.

## CHAPTER 7: TENDING TO OUR GARDENS

1. "Our Mission at UPS," n.d., https://unitedplantsavers.org/40-our-mission-ups.

2. "Códice de la Cruz-Badiano, Parte II," *Arqueología Mexicana* 51 (2013), 21.

3. "Códice de la Cruz-Badiano," 15.

4. *Atlas de las plantas de la medicina tradicional Mexicana*, s.v. "Mirto," Biblioteca Digital de la Medicina Tradicional Mexicana, accessed September 28, 2021, www.medicinatradicionalmexicana.unam.mx/apmtm/termino.php?l=3&t=salvia-microphylla.

5. Nareni Pliego Osorio, *Catálogo de plantas medicinales del Jardín Botánico del Instituto de Biología* (tesis de diplomado, TlahuiEdu, Ciudad de México, 2011), 60–61.

6. Aida Guerra Falcón, *Medicina tradicional Doña Queta y el legado de los habitantes de Las Nubes* (self-published, Oaxaca, Mexico, 2009), 140.

7. *Atlas de las plantas de la medicina tradicional Mexicana*, s.v. "Lana o Salvia," Biblioteca Digital de la Medicina Tradicional Mexicana, accessed September 28, 2021, http://www.medicinatradicionalmexicana.unam.mx/apmtm/termino.php?l=3&t=salvia-leucantha.

8. Leslie Gardner, *Life in the Medicine: A Guide to Growing and Harvesting Herbs for Medicine Making* (Sebastopol, CA: Emerald Earth, 2008), 85.

9. Joie Davidow, *Infusions of Healing: A Treasury of Mexican-American Herbal Remedies* (New York: Simon & Schuster, 1999), 118.

10. *Atlas de las plantas de la medicina tradicional Mexicana*, s.v. "Estafiate," Biblioteca Digital de la Medicina Tradicional Mexicana, accessed September 28, 2021, http://www.medicinatradicionalmexicana.unam.mx/apmtm/termino.php?l=3&t=artemisia-ludoviciana.

11. Eliseo "Cheo" Torres, *Curanderismo: The Art of Traditional Medicine without Borders* (Dubuque, IA: Kendall Hunt, 2017), 26.

12. *Atlas de las Plantas*, "Estafiate."

13. Eliseo "Cheo" Torres, *Healing with Herbs and Rituals: A Mexican Tradition* (Albuquerque: University of New Mexico Press, 2006), 15.

14. Falcón, 148–49.

15. Gardner, 98.

16. Falcón, 226.

17. Davidow, 93.

18. "Tagetes erecta - L.," Plants for a Future, n.d., https://pfaf.org/user/Plant.aspx?LatinName=Tagetes+erecta.

19. *Atlas de las plantas de la medicina tradicional Mexicana*, s.v. "Cempasúchil o flor de muerto," Biblioteca Digital de la Medicina Tradicional Mexicana, accessed September 28, 2021, http://www.medicinatradicionalmexicana.unam.mx/apmtm/termino.php?l=3&t=cempasuchil-flor-muerto.

20. Falcón, 127–28.

21. *Atlas de las plantas*, "Cempasúchil o flor de muerto."

22. Patrisia Gonzales, *Red Medicine: Traditional Indigenous Rites of Birthing and Healing* (Tucson: University of Arizona Press, 2012), chap. 1.

23. Dora Sierra Carrillo, *El demonio anda suelto: El poder de la Cruz de Pericón* (Ciudad de México: Instituto Nacional de Antropología e Historia, 2019), 38.

24. Edelmira Linares Mazari, Robert Arthur Bye Boettler, and Beatriz Flores, *Plantas medicinales de México: Usos, remedios y tradiciones* (Ciudad de México: Instituto de Biología, Universidad Nacional Autonoma de México, 1999).

25. Gonzales, chap. 1.

26. Carrillo, 39.

27. Jaime Trujillo, "An Experience with La Abuelita's Favorite Remedy: The Uses of *Tagetes lucida* (pericón)," *Journal of the American Herbalist Guild* 15, no. 1 (Spring 2017), 13–18.

28. Falcón, 219.

29. Falcón, 219.

30. Trujillo, 13–18.

31. Gardner, 99.

32. *Atlas de plantas de la medicina tradicional Mexicana*, s.v. "Ruda," Biblioteca Digital de la Medicina Tradicional Mexicana, accessed September 28, 2021, http://www.medicinatradicionalmexicana.unam.mx/apmtm/termino.php?l=3&t=ruta-graveolens.

33. Falcón, 229.

34. Gonzales, chap 1.

35. Notes from Traditional Medicine without Borders class, University of New Mexico Albuquerque, organized by Eliseo "Cheo" Torres, taught by Doris Ortiz, 2011.

36. Rick Kurtz, "How to Grow Peruvian Pepper Trees," *SFGATE*, n.d., https://homeguides.sfgate.com/grow-peruvian-pepper-trees-73271.html.

37. Eliseo "Cheo" Torres with Timothy L. Sawyer Jr., *Curandero: A Life in Mexican Folk Healing* (Albuquerque: University of New Mexico Press, 2005).

38. *Atlas de las plantas de la medicina tradicional Mexicana*, s.v. "Pirul," Biblioteca Digital de la Medicina Tradicional Mexicana, accessed September 29, 2021, http://www.medicinatradicionalmexicana.unam.mx/apmtm/termino.php?l=3&t=schinus-molle.

39. *Atlas de las plantas*, "Pirul."

40. Notes from Traditional Medicine without Borders class.

41. Gardner, 59.

42. Osorio, *Catálogo de plantas medicinales*.

43. Karen Knipping, Johan Garssen, and Belinda van't Land, "An Evaluation of the Inhibitory Effects against Rotavirus Infection of Edible Plant Extracts," *Virology Journal* 9, no. 137 (2012), https://doi.org/10.1186/1743-422X-9-137; Akram Astani, Mojdeh Heidary Navid, and Paul Schnitzler, "Attachment and Penetration of Acyclovir-Resistant Herpes Simplex Virus Are Inhibited by *Melissa officinalis* Extract," *Phytotherapy Research* 28, no.10 (2014): 1547–52, https://doi.org/10.1002/ptr.5166.

## CHAPTER 9: NOURISHMENT: HERBAL TONICS AND FOOD AS MEDICINE

1. Leslie Gardner, *Life in the Medicine: A Guide to Growing and Harvesting Herbs for Medicine Making* (Sebastopol, CA: Emerald Earth, 2008), 87.
2. Laban K. Rutto, Yixiang Xu, Elizabeth Ramirez, and Michael Brandt, "Mineral Properties and Dietary Value of Raw and Processed Stinging Nettle (*Urtica dioica* L.)," *International Journal of Food Science* 2013, article ID 857120. https://doi.org/10.1155/2013/857120.
3. Aida Guerra Falcón, *Medicina tradicional Doña Queta y el legado de los habitantes de Las Nubes* (self-published, Oaxaca, Mexico, 2009), 215.
4. W. J. Rayment, "The History of Oregano," http://www.indepthinfo.com /oregano/history.shtml (site discontinued).
5. Falcón, 214.
6. Joie Davidow, *Infusions of Healing: A Treasury of Mexican-American Herbal Remedies* (New York: Simon & Schuster, 1999), 155.
7. Gretchen Heber, "How to Grow Mexican Oregano," *Gardener's Path*, March 9, 2020, https://gardenerspath.com/plants/herbs/grow-mexican-oregano.
8. Francisco Hernández, in *The Mexican Treasury: The Writings of Dr. Francisco Hernández*, ed. Simon Varey, trans. Rafael Chabrán, Cynthia L. Chamberlin, and Simon Varey (Stanford, CA: Stanford University Press, 2000), 118.
9. Hernández, 156; Charles W. Kane, *Herbal Medicine of the American Southwest* (n.p.: Lincoln Town Press, 2006), 87.
10. Gardner, 38.
11. Gretchen Herber, "How to Grow and Use Epazote Herb," *Gardener's Path*, October 9, 2019, https://gardenerspath.com/plants/herbs/grow-epazote.
12. *Atlas de las plantas de la medicina tradicional Mexicana*, s.v. "Epazote," Biblioteca Digital de la Medicina Tradicional Mexicana, accessed September 28, 2021, http://www.medicinatradicionalmexicana.unam.mx/apmtm /termino.php?l=3&t=epazote.
13. Kraig H. Kraft, Cecil H. Brown, Gary P. Nabhan, Eike Luedeling, José de Jesús Luna Ruiz, Geo Coppens d'Eeckenbrugge, Robert J. Hijmans, and Paul Gepts, "Multiple Lines of Evidence for the Origin of Domesticated Chili Pepper, *Capsicum annuum*, in Mexico," *Proceedings of the National Academy of Sciences* 111, no. 17 (2014): 6165–70, https://doi.org/10.1073 /pnas.1308933111; Linda Perry and Kent V. Flannery, "Precolumbian Use

of Chili Peppers in the Valley of Oaxaca, Mexico," Proceedings of the National Academy of Sciences 104, no. 29 (2007): 11905–09, https://doi.org/10.1073/pnas.0704936104.

14. Falcón, 135.

15. Ryusuke Nishio, Hanuna Tamano, Hiroki Morioka, Azusa Takeuchi, and Atsushi Takeda, "Intake of Heated Leaf Extract of *Coriandrum sativum* Contributes to Resistance to Oxidative Stress via Decreases in Heavy Metal Concentrations in the Kidney," *Plant Foods for Human Nutrition* 74, no. 2 (2019): 204–09, https://doi.org/10.1007/s11130-019-00720-2.

16. Georgia Schäfer and Catherine H. Kaschula, "The Immunomodulation and Anti-Inflammatory Effects of Garlic Organosulfur Compounds in Cancer Chemoprevention," *Anti-Cancer Agents in Medicinal Chemistry* 14, no. 2 (2014): 233–40, https://doi.org/10.2174/18715206113136660370.

17. Rodrigo Arreola, Saray Quintero-Fabián, Rocío Ivette López-Roa, Enrique Octavio Flores-Gutiérrez, Juan Pablo Reyes-Grajeda, Lucrecia Carrera-Quintanar, and Daniel Ortuño-Sahagún, "Immunomodulation and Anti-Inflammatory Effects of Garlic Compounds," *Journal of Immunology Research* 2015, https://doi.org/10.1155/2015/401630.

18. "Growing Onions," *Old Farmer's Almanac*, n.d., https://www.almanac.com/plant/onions.

19. Molly Knudsen, "What Makes Onions So Healthy? It's Quercetin," *Metagenics Blog*, August 26, 2020, https://blog.metagenics.com/post/2020/08/26/what-makes-onions-so-healthy-its-quercetin.

20. Holly L. Nicastro, Sharon A. Ross, and John A. Milner, "Garlic and Onions: Their Cancer Prevention Properties," *Cancer Prevention Research* 8, no. 3 (2015): 181–89, https://doi.org/10.1158/1940-6207.CAPR-14-0172; "Onion Health Research," National Onion Association, n.d., https://www.onions-usa.org/all-about-onions/onion-health-research.

**CHAPTER 10: ENERGY AND BOUNDARIES**

1. Sergio Magaña (Ocelocoyotl), *2012–2021—The Dawn of the Sixth Sun: The Path of Quetzalcoatl* (Giaveno, Italy: BlossomingBooks, 2012), 22.

2. Patricia Chicueyi Coatl, personal correspondance with the author, March 20, 2021.

3. Alfredo López Austin, *The Human Body and Ideology: Concepts of the Ancient Nahuas*, vol. 2, trans. Thelma Ortiz de Montellano and Bernard Ortiz de Montellano (Salt Lake City: University of Utah Press, 1988).

4. Dora Sierra Carrillo, *El demonio anda suelto: El poder de la Cruz de Pericón* (Ciudad de México: Instituto Nacional de Antropología e Historia, 2019), 46.
5. Magaña, 150.
6. Magaña, 150.
7. Magaña, 150.
8. Carrillo, 45.
9. Carrillo, 45.
10. Carrillo, 45.
11. David Carrasco, Scott Sessions, and Eduardo Matos Moctezuma, *Moctezuma's Mexico: Visions of the Aztec World*, rev. ed. (Boulder: University Press of Colorado, 2003).
12. Frances Karttunen, *An Analytical Dictionary of Nahuatl* (Norman: University of Oklahoma Press, 1992), 98.
13. Gonzales, 204–5.
14. Magaña, 33.
15. James Maffie, "Aztec Philosophy," *Internet Encyclopedia of Philosophy*, n.d., https://iep.utm.edu/aztec.
16. Carrillo, 47.
17. Patrisia Gonzales, *Red Medicine: Traditional Indigenous Rites of Birthing and Healing* (Tucson: University of Arizona Press, 2012), chap. 1.
18. Gonzales, chap. 1.
19. Gonzales, chap. 1.

## CHAPTER 11: DANCING WITH LOS AIRES

1. Estela Román, *Nuestra medicina: De los remedíos para el aire y los remedíos para el alma* (Bloomington, IN: Palibrio, 2012).
2. Anna Joyce, *The Sixth Sun: The Spiritual Path and Practice of Mexican-American Curanderismo* (PhD diss., California Institute of Integral Studies, San Francisco, 2011), 300; Román, *Nuestra medicina*.
3. Joyce, 13.

## CHAPTER 12: CLEANSING OURSELVES: LIMPIAS AND BAÑOS

1. Notes from Limpias, class taught by Laurencio López Núñez, Sol Collective, Sacramento, CA, June 2019. Translated from the Spanish.
2. Patrisia Gonzales, *Red Medicine: Traditional Indigenous Rites of Birthing and Healing* (Tucson: University of Arizona Press, 2012), chap. 1.

3.  Gonzales, chap. 1.

4.  Dora Sierra Carrillo, *El demonio anda suelto: El poder de la Cruz de Pericón* (Ciudad de México: Instituto Nacional de Antropología e Historia, 2019), 48.

5.  Carrillo, 45.

6.  Patricia Chicueyi Coatl, "Sahumador," *Calmecac Huey Papalotl* (unpublished class reader, 2014), 68.

7.  Eliseo "Cheo" Torres, *Curanderismo: The Art of Traditional Medicine without Borders* (Dubuque, IA: Kendall Hunt, 2017), 26.

8.  Chichueyi Coatl, "Sahumador," 69.

9.  Serife Karagozoglu, Filiz Tekyasar, and Figen Alp Yilmaz, "Effects of Music Therapy and Guided Visual Imagery on Chemotherapy-Induced Anxiety and Nausea–Vomiting," *Journal of Clinical Nursing* 22, nos. 1–2 (2013): 39–50, https://doi.org/10.1111/jocn.12030; Andrew Rossetti, Manjeet Chadha, B. Nelson Torres, Jae K. Lee, Donald Hylton, Joanne V. Loewy, and Louis B. Harrison, "The Impact of Music Therapy on Anxiety in Cancer Patients Undergoing Simulation for Radiation Therapy," *International Journal of Radiation Oncology, Biology, Physics* 99, no. 1 (2017): 103–10, https://doi.org/10.1016/j.ijrobp.2017.05.003.

10. M. Gómez Gallego and J. Gómez García, "Music Therapy and Alzheimer's Disease: Cognitive, Psychological, and Behavioural Effects," *Neurologia* 32, no. 5 (2017): 300–08, English, Spanish, https://doi.org/10.1016/j.nrl.2015.12.003; Daisy Fancourt, Rosie Perkins, Sara Ascenso, Livia A. Carvalho, Andrew Steptoe, and Aaron Williamon, "Effects of Group Drumming Interventions on Anxiety, Depression, Social Resilience and Inflammatory Immune Response among Mental Health Service Users," *PloS ONE* 11, no. 3 (2016): e0151136, https://doi.org/10.1371/journal.pone.0151136.

11. Robert Lawrence Friedman, *The Healing Power of the Drum* (Reno, NV: White Cliffs Media, 2000).

12. Gonzales, chap. 4.

13. Sergio Magaña, *The Real Toltec Prophecies: How the Aztec Calendar Predicted Modern-Day Events and Reveals a Pathway to a New Era of Humankind* (Carlsbad, CA: Hay House, 2020), chap. 8.

14. Gonzales, chap. 4.

15. Silvia Trejo, "Xochiquétzal y Tlazoltéotl. Diosas mexicanas del amor y la sexualidad," *Arqueología Mexicana*, no. 87: 18–25, https://arqueologiamexicana.mx/mexico-antiguo/xochiquetzal-y-tlazolteotl-diosas-mexicas-del-amor-y-la-sexualidad.

## CHAPTER 13: LA MEDICINA OF DREAMS

1. Eleanor Barron-Druckrey, *A Dream Map to the Sixth Sun: Restoring Harmony and Balance to Our Lives* (self-published: Xlibris, 2017), 13–16.

2. Sergio Magaña, *The Toltec Secret: Dreaming Practices of the Ancient Mexicans* (Carlsbad, CA: Hay House, 2014), 39.

3. Magaña, *Toltec Secret.*

4. Magaña, *Toltec Secret.*

5. Leslie Gardner, *Life in the Medicine: A Guide to Growing and Harvesting Herbs for Medicine Making* (Sebastopol, CA: Emerald Earth, 2008), 47.

6. Barron-Druckrey, 13–16.

# Image Credits

For all images not in the public domain, all reasonable attempts were made to locate the copyright holders for the material published in this book. If you believe you may be one of them, please contact Heyday and the publisher will include appropriate acknowledgment in subsequent editions of this book.

Images credited "from Köhler" are from Hermann Adolph Köhler, *Köhler's Medizinal-Pflanzen*, 1887, public domain, accessed at Biodiversity Heritage Library, https://www.biodiversitylibrary.org/bibliography/623.

Page viii: Virgin of Guadalupe (Virgen de Guadalupe). By Manuel de Arellano, 1691, oil painting on canvas, Los Angeles County Museum of Art, Los Angeles, CA. Available at Wikimedia Commons, https://commons.wikimedia.org/wiki/File:Manuel_de_Arellano_-_Virgin_of_Guadalupe_(Virgen_de_Guadalupe)_-_Google_Art_Project.jpg.

Page xii: Marigold. From Basilius Besler, *Hortus Eystettensis*, first published 1613.

Page 2: Bundle. From iStock, number 157560196.

Page 2: Copalera. By Mia Altar.

Page 7: The author. By Vaschelle André.

Page 16: Trudy Robles. By Sofia Robles Castillo.

Page 21: Dandelion. From Köhler.

Page 25: Botanical drawing. From Martín de la Cruz, *Códice de la Cruz-Badiano*, 1552, National Institute of Anthropology and History in Mexico City, Mexico.

Page 26: Botanical drawings. From Martín de la Cruz, *Códice de la Cruz-Badiano*, 1552, National Institute of Anthropology and History in Mexico City, Mexico.

Page 28 The Aztec day sign *coatl* (snake). From the Codex Magliabechiano, mid sixteenth century, Biblioteca Nazionale Centrale, Florence, Italy. Available at Wikimedia Commons, https://en.wiktionary.org/wiki/coatl#/media/File:Coatl.jpg.

Page 31: Reishi mushroom. From iStock, ID 1330220735.

Page 36: Maria Miranda. By Lozen Miranda Brightman.

Page 40: Marigold (*Tagetes erecta*). Available at https://www.pinterest.com/pin/4566228496901 35848.

Page 43: *Prunella vulgaris*. By Jan Christiaan Sepp for Jan Kops et al., *Flora Batava: Afbeelding en Beschrijving van Nederlandsche Gewassen*, Vol. 1 (Amsterdam: J. C. Sepp en Zoon, 1800). Available at Kurt Stüber's Online Library, http://www.biolib.de/batava/band1/high /IMG_8347.html.

Page 50: Marcela Sabin. By Ezekiel Mansilla.

Page 52:    Rosemary. From Köhler.

Page 60:    Dandelion. From Köhler.

Page 68:    Candice Rose Valenzuela. By Candice Rose Valenzuela.

Page 70:    Tobacco flower. From Köhler.

Page 80:    Teotihuacan engraving, Mexico City. From Shutterstock, ID 1738656809.

Page 88:    Antique rusty milagros heart. From iStock, ID 1316868943.

Page 90:    Patricia Chicueyi Coatl, by Brooke Anderson.

Page 94:    Chamomile. From Köhler.

Page 97:    Nasturtium. From Shutterstock, ID 126332032.

Page 100:   Koi. From Creative Market.

Page 103:   Cacao. From Manuel Blanco, *Flora de Filipinas, Gran edicion* (Manila, 1877). Available at Wikimedia Commons, https://commons.wikimedia.org/wiki/File:Theobroma_cacao_Blanco_clean.jpg.

Page 113:   Tobacco. From Etienne Denise, *Flore d'Amérique*, (Paris: Chez Gihaut Freres, 1843), Lu-Esther T. Mertz Library at New York Botanical Garden. Available at Biodiversity Heritage Library, https://www.biodiversitylibrary.org/item/185335.

Page 114:   Berenice Dimas. By Heather Bejar (makeup by Linda Yoon).

Page 118:   Salvia. From Köhler.

Page 121:   Garden. By Batul True Heart.

Page 122:   Salvia. From Köhler.

Page 122:   *Salvia microphylla*. By First Light, 2008. Available at Wikimedia Commons, https://commons.wikimedia.org/wiki/File:Salvia_microphylla_neurepia.jpg.

Page 122:   *Salvia greggii*. By Ray Mathews, 2013. Available at Wildflower Center Digital Library, https://www.wildflower.org/gallery/result.php?id_image=38136.

Page 123:   Mexican sage, *Salvia leucantha*. From iStock, ID 543483536.

Page 124:   Peppermint. From Köhler.

Page 125:   Spearmint. From Köhler.

Page 126:   Mugwort. From Köhler.

Page 128:   Rosemary. From Köhler.

Page 130:   Marigold. Available at https://www.pinterest.com/pin/456622849690135848.

Page 130:   *Tagetes erecta*. By Bishnu Sarangi, 2016. Available at Pixabay, https://pixabay.com/photos/flower-marigold-orange-field-plant-1659660.

Page 131:   *Tagetes lucida*. From Shutterstock, ID 49262248.

Page 132:   *Tagetes lemmonii*. From iStock, ID 883774486.

Page 134:   Rue. From Köhler.

Page 136:   Pirul. From Rare Book Division, New York Public Library, "Schinus molle = Mollé à folioles dentées. [Brazilian pepper tree, Peruvian music tree, California pepper tree etc.]," Available at New York Public Library Digital Collections, https://digitalcollections.nypl.org/items/510d47dc-9235-a3d9-e040-e00a18064a99.

Page 137:   Elderberry. From Köhler.

Page 139:  Chamomile. From Köhler.

Page 140:  Melissa/lemon balm. From Köhler.

Page 142:  RaheNi Gonzalez. By RaheNi Gonzalez.

Page 146:  Elderberry. From Köhler.

Page 154:  Red clover. From Otto Wilhelm Thomé, *Flora von Deutschland, Österreich und der Schweiz*, (Gera-Untermhaus, Verlag von Fr. Eugen Köhler, 1885–1905). Available at Kurt Stüber's Online Library, http://www.biolib.de/thome/thome_flora_von_deutschland_tafeln.pdf.

Page 155:  Tincture bottle. From iStock, ID 480050651.

Page 166:  Batul True Heart. By Batul True Heart.

Page 168:  Pepper. From Köhler.

Page 170:  Stinging nettle. From Otto Wilhelm Thomé, *Flora von Deutschland, Österreich und der Schweiz*, (Gera-Untermhaus: Verlag von Fr. Eugen Köhler, 1885–1905). Available at Kurt Stüber's Online Library, http://www.biolib.de/thome/thome_flora_von_deutschland_tafeln.pdf.

Page 171:  Wild oat (*Avena sativa*). From Friedrich Losch, *Kräuterbuch: Unsere Heilpflanzen in Wort und Bild, Zweite Auflage*, (Esslingen: J. F. Schreiber, 1905) t. 6, fig. 1. Missouri Botanical Garden, Peter H. Raven Library. Available at Biodiversity Heritage Library, https://www.biodiversitylibrary.org/bibliography/39396.

Page 173:  Mediterranean oregano. From John Stephenson and James Morss Churchill, *Medical botany: Comprising a popular and scientific account of poisonous vegetables indigenous to Great Britain, vol. 3* (London: John Churchill, 1836), plate 131. Available at Freepik, https://www.freepik.com/free-photo/oregano-origanum-vulgare-illustration-from-medical-botany-1836_3533341.htm.

Page 174:  Mexican oregano (*Lippia graveolens*). By Dick Culbert, 2013. Available at Wikimedia Commons, https://commons.wikimedia.org/wiki/File:Lippia_graveolens,_known_as_Mexican_Oregano_(11628265214).jpg.

Page 174:  Monarda. From iStock, ID 1331812421.

Page 175:  Epazote. From Manuel Blanco, *Flora de Filipinas, Gran edicion* (Manila, 1877). Available at Wikimedia Commons, https://commons.wikimedia.org/wiki/File:Dysphania_ambrosioides_Blanco1.69-original.png.

Page 176:  Pepper. From Köhler.

Page 177:  Coriander. From Köhler.

Page 178:  Garlic. Available at Instituto Químico Biológico, https://www.iqb.es/cbasicas/farma/farma06/plantas/pa13.htm.

Page 179:  Onion. From Otto Wilhelm Thomé, *Flora von Deutschland, Österreich und der Schweiz* (Gera-Untermhaus: Verlag von Fr. Eugen Köhler, 1885–1905). Available at Kurt Stüber's Online Library, http://www.biolib.de/thome/thome_flora_von_deutschland_tafeln.pdf.

Page 186:  Ginger. From Etienne Denise, *Flore d'Amérique*, (Paris: Chez Gihaut Freres, 1843) 149, Lu-Esther T. Mertz Library at New York Botanical Garden. Available at Biodiversity Heritage Library, https://www.biodiversitylibrary.org/item/185335.

Page 188: Sandra M. Pacheco. By Diego Aquino.

Page 190: Yarrow. From Köhler.

Page 200: Yarrow. From Köhler.

Page 201: Tobacco. From Otto Wilhelm Thomé, *Flora von Deutschland, Österreich und der Schweiz* (Gera-Untermhaus: Verlag von Fr. Eugen Köhler, 1885–1905). Available at Kurt Stüber's Online Library, http://www.biolib.de/thome/thome_flora_von_deutschland_tafeln.pdf.

Page 204: Brenda Salgado. By Ramin Rahimian.

Page 208: Sunflower. From Köhler.

Page 209: The Aztec day sign *ehecatl* (wind). From the Codex Magliabechiano, mid sixteenth century, Biblioteca Nazionale Centrale, Florence, Italy. Available at Wikimedia Commons, https://commons.wikimedia.org/wiki/Aztec_glyphs#/media/File:Ehecatl2.jpg.

Page 218: Altar. By Batul True Heart.

Page 230: Angela Raquel Aguilar. By Alejandra Olguin.

Page 234: Rose, circa 1883. Available at the Graphics Fairy, https://thegraphicsfairy.com/10-free-vintage-roses-images.

Page 241: Herb bundle. By Batul True Heart.

Page 251: Baño. By Batul True Heart.

Page 252: Marigold. From Köhler.

Page 254: Alejandra Olguin. By Jacinto Mingura.

Page 256: California poppy. Available at Hollander's, https://hollanders.com/products/florentine-print-california-poppy?variant=30286114193462.

Page 259: Scullcap. From Charles Frederick Millspaugh, *American Medicinal Plants*, (New York: Boericke & Tafel, 1887). NCSU Libraries. Available at Biodiversity Heritage Library, https://www.biodiversitylibrary.org/bibliography/37663.

Page 260: Passionflower. From iStock, ID 500278187.

Page 261: California poppy. Available at Hollander's, https://hollanders.com/products/florentine-print-california-poppy?variant=30286114193462.

Page 263: Mugwort. From Köhler.

Page 264: Lavender. From Köhler.

Page 274: Eleanor "Ellie" Barron-Druckrey. By Randall R. Druckrey.

Page 292: The author. By Vaschelle André.

# About the Author

Atava Garcia Swiecicki is guided by the plants, her dreams, and her Mexican, Polish, Hungarian, and Diné ancestors. She received a BA in feminist studies from Stanford University and a master's degree from the Indigenous Mind Program at Naropa University Oakland. Atava has studied healing arts extensively for over thirty years and has been mentored by herbalists, curanderas, and traditional knowledge keepers. She works as a clinical herbalist and teacher. She is the founder of the Ancestral Apothecary School of Herbal, Folk, and Indigenous Medicine on unceded Lisjan Ohlone territory in Oakland, and she currently lives in unceded Tewa Pueblo territory in Albuquerque. Her personal website is ancestralapothecary.com, and the website for her school is ancestralapothecaryschool.com.

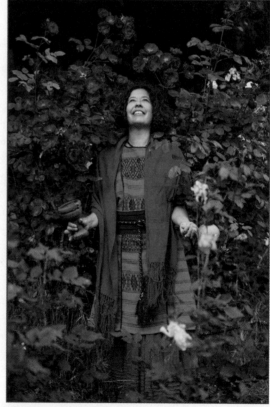

Photo by Vaschelle André